Rheumatology in the United Kingdom. 50 years of progress

Allan St John Dixon

Rheumatology in the United Kingdom- 50 years of progress

Copyright © 2000

Published in the United Kingdom by Allan St John Dixon. OBE, MD, FRCP

Printed by Troutbeck Press, Penryn, Cornwall

ISBN No 0-9537628-0-7

Table of contents

In 1952 the Nuffield Foundation awarded me a Fellowship to study rheumatology with Walter Bauer in Boston. So when the Oliver Bird Fund of the Foundation asked me in late 1997 to write a history of rheumatology to mark the 50th anniversary of the Fund in September 1998, I could not but accept. The brief was a history of UK rheumatology as a whole, not just a history of the Oliver Bird Fund. A synopsis was produced and agreed. The main narrative would start at 1948 but an earlier chapter would introduce this by recalling the scene in the first half of the century. The history would be about 40,000 words long. Time was short but it looked possible.

In the event the history ran to over 80,000 words and this together with unforeseen delays made it impossible to meet the intended deadline, a setback that provided an opportunity for an extensive revision of the text and to take the story up to 1999. Readers in the new millennium can look back at the remarkable changes that have taken place in over 50 years of the old one.

This is a *'was then, is now'* sort of history rather than a year by year almanac of events. Many people, some of them themselves recipients of financial support from the Oliver Bird Fund and/or from the Arthritis Research Campaign, have helped generously with information and archival material, but any errors, opinions or omissions are mine.

A. S. Dixon.

I am glad to preface this grand achievement by Allan Dixon. It needed to be done and to be done well. His story of the development and fruition of rheumatology in the United Kingdom (UK) during the last five decades has covered an era of great advances in this previously somewhat neglected subject. As in other countries including the United States of America the growth of rheumatology has been led and stimulated against a background of enormous and world-wide changes in science generally and in biology and medicine in particular.

The year 1948 was the *Annus Mirabilis* of rheumatology. It had already begun to separate from Physical Medicine and Spa therapy with which it had traditionally been associated and to join General Medicine as a respected speciality in its own right.

The author starts with a brief account of the pioneers who initiated this breakaway process. As part of this, the International Society of Medical Hydrology set up in 1921 became the International League against Rheumatism (ILAR) in 1928, reappearing after the war.

It was in 1948 that Nye Bevan, introducing the UK National Health Service, promised "Medicine for all, regardless of status or ability to pay." Those early years saw the introduction of post-graduate medical education, controlled clinical trials, the recognition of paediatric rheumatology, the start of surgical joint replacements for osteoarthritis, the introduction of cortisone and adrenocorticotrophic hormone, the successful use of uricosuric drugs for gout and new painkillers starting with phenylbutazone. But most important were the antibiotics starting with the suphonamides, penicillin and the anti-tuberculous drugs. Many of these advances had applications in rheumatology. Much current immunological research can trace its origins back to the recognition at that time of the Lupus Erythematosus (LE) and Rheumatoid Arthritis (RA) factors.

It was in this heady atmosphere of startling discoveries that Allan Dixon began his medical career in Rheumatology and became an integral part of that advance-in research, in clinical and epidemiological medicine. History from the Inside!

As consultant in London and later Bath he contributed research papers (200 publications) and initiated REMEDI (the Rehabilitation and Medical Research Trust), the Society for Back Pain Research and the Research Institute for the Care of the Elderly. On the social side he founded the special interest associations, the National Ankylosing Spondylitis Society and more recently The National Osteoporosis Society. He has served as Medical Secretary of the Arthritis and Rheumatism Council and as Secretary-General of the European League against Rheumatism.

To complement this study of advances in these five decades he has added a survey of the old and new centres established in the NHS for the study and treatment of the rheumatic diseases.

The book lists some of the successes, failures and future trends in rheumatology. Most importantly it contains a history of a patient born in 1924 with experience of all the problems that severe rheumatoid arthritis can bring over 33 years, to remind us of the centre of all our activities.

"History is the essence of innumerable biographies" wrote Thomas Carlyle. And so is clinical medicine.

EGL Bywaters, Beaconsfield, June 1999

Chapter 1.
The Setting before 1948

Chronic rheumatic diseases before 1948 had a low priority in London teaching hospitals. Patients suffering from them were regarded as bed-blockers and not often admitted. Outside London patients went to the Spa hospitals. In London there were two outpatient rheumatism Institutes, the Kensington Institute for Rheumatic Diseases, that did not survive post-war reorganisation, and the British Red Cross Institute, opened in 1930 at Peto Place, that did.

Under the Local Government Act of 1929, the early 'Poor Law' hospitals had been taken over and transformed by the London County Council that had in 1937 established a rheumatology service at St Stephen's Hospital in Chelsea under Drs Philip Ellman and Francis Bach. In 1938 at the Middlesex Hospital Dr WSC Copeman had expanded his paediatric clinic to take adults as well as children with chronic arthritis. Elsewhere in London arthritis patients might be referred to physical medicine specialists, some of whom, as at St Mary Abbot's Hospital in Kensington, were little more than signposts to their physiotherapy departments. Aspirin and gold preparations were the main drugs used. Some doctors still believed focal sepsis to be the cause of rheumatoid arthritis and certain London consultants found they had a profitable little earner in administering autogenous vaccines prepared from nasopharyngeal washings and made for them by Sir Almoth Wright at St Mary's Hospital. This treatment was centred on the Charterhouse Clinics in London and persisted long after its medical value was debunked. There were other, mainly London, consultants with a wider vision.

Father Figures of modern Rheumatology..

'The Dark Ages of Rheumatology' is how some have described the treatment of rheumatism patients pre-1948, and particularly pre-war. Such research as had been done was mainly observational and descriptive. Bogus treatments abounded (as, of course, they still do today). John Hilton's famous book *Rest and Pain* which expounded the curative powers of rest had been a powerful antidote to the interference by both orthodox and heterodox practitioners in the natural healing processes. But his principles were followed too blindly in the rheumatic diseases, forgetting that healing of diseases of the locomotor apparatus requires some movement to conserve function. Rheumatoid arthritis sufferers were put to bed only to emerge with the classic 'bed deformities' (Figure 1.1). Ankylosing spondylitis treated by orthopaedic surgeons on the lines previously used for tuberculosis of the spine meant Swain's corsets or plaster body shells, which turned patients into virtual statues. Radiotherapy relieved pain in ankylosing spondylitis but increased the risk of leukaemia, Bowen's disease and delayed radiation damage to the spinal cord. Gout was treated by colchicine, but one had to take it to the point of diarrhoea for it to be effective and it did nothing to prevent urate accumulation in the body. But even if it was a dark night for rheumatology, dark nights have bright stars.

Amongst these was Will Copeman (1900-1970) (Figure 1.2), whose personal scientific contributions to rheumatology were minimal yet whose influence on the emergence of British rheumatology as a Specialty in its own right is difficult to

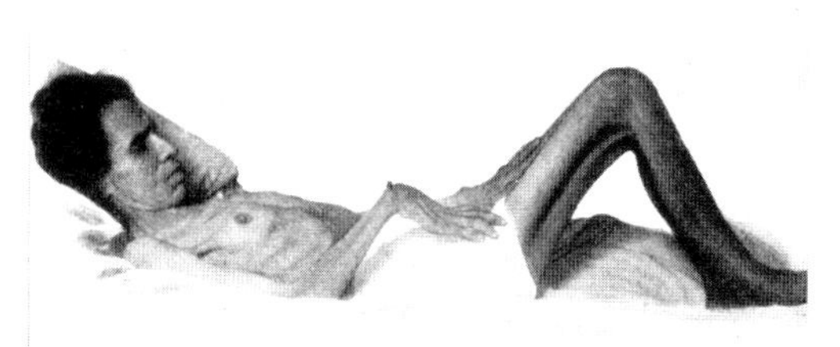

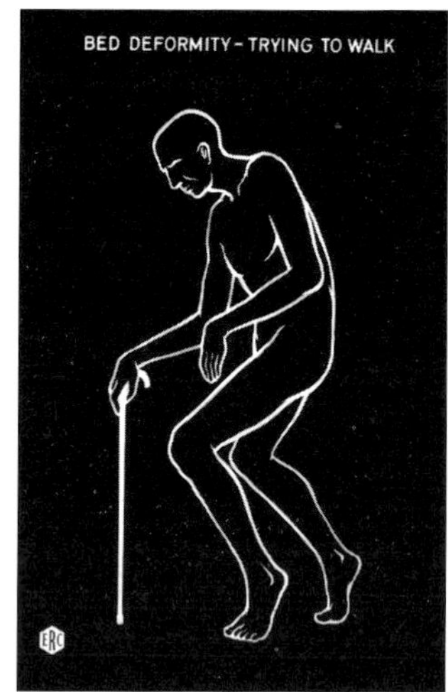

Figure 1.1. a The Bed Deformity. A neglected and bed-bound rheumatoid arthritis patient, showing flexion contractures of the neck,hips and knees, dropped ankles and wrists. 1.1.b Trying to walk.

overestimate. He took a leading role in every significant development in the early days of UK rheumatology (see box).

He was a complex personality and the many people who knew him or wrote about him saw him in as many different ways. He has been variously called the Father of British Rheumatology and the biggest rheumatological 'fixer' of all time. He had the vision in pre-war days to see that the treatment of chronic arthritis had to be wrested from the traditional and empirical methods available in the hospital physical medicine departments and spa hospitals. He inspired diligent loyalty in those who worked for him and a sense of bitterness in some of them when he failed, so it must have appeared, to back them for an appropriate job when they left him. A personal rift with Francis Bach became a chasm that 50 years later continued to divide the Arthritis and Rheumatism Council (ARC), *later called the Arthritis Research Campaign and previously known as the Empire Rheumatism Council* (ERC), from the British Rheumatism Association, *(later renamed Arthritis Care),* at headquarters level, despite their common interests and sometimes mutual cooperation at local support group level. However by 1999 the two organisations did collaborate in a number of ways, particularly in the provision of educational materials. Both became members of the British League against Rheumatism. This enabled them to present a common face to other specialties, to governmental departments and to rheumatology in other countries.

To some Copeman was austere and unapproachable, others saw the twinkle in his eye. Dr Beric Wright, at one time connected to the Institute of Directors, pronounced him arrogant at a committee meeting of the Back Pain Association. But as the appreciation of him by Porritt and Hart (1972) makes clear, "He was seldom entirely sure he was in the right, would ask others for their opinion and ....usually acted upon it". This occasional loss of self-assurance showed itself when he was asked to lecture to the students at the Postgraduate Medical School. The rheumatology staff were pointedly told they were not expected to attend.

Dr John Glyn who knew him well remembers how he was called to Copeman's consulting rooms to be interviewed for the position of co-ordinater of the United Kingdom trial of Cortisone versus Aspirin in rheumatoid arthritis. His

WSC Copeman, CBE, TD, JP, MA, MD, FRCP. 1900-1970

Consultant Physician, The Middlesex Hospital. Son of Dr S Monckton Copeman

1918 Second Lieutenant, (Coldstream Guards).

1919-25 Medical student at St Thomas' Medical School.

1922-32 He would have been aware of the four reports by J A Glover to the Minister of Health, entitled 'Chronic Arthritis with Special Reference to Provision of Treatment.'

1925 Graduated. After junior hospital appointments he was in 1937 appointed consultant physician to the Hospital of St John and Elizabeth and paediatrician to the West London Hospital. There he set up a children's rheumatism clinic which soon began to accept adults with rheumatic diseases.

1933 Royal College of Physicians, Special Commission on Rheumatic Diseases.

1936 Empire Rheumatism Council (ERC) formed, its committee included Copeman taking a lead under the chairmanship of Lord Horder.

1936 3rd March, Matthew Ray chaired a meeting of six doctors including Copeman at Peto Place to form the 'Clinical Group for the Study of the Rheumatic Disorders'. The following year it was named the Heberden Society and thrown open to a limit of 100 doctors.

1937 Copeman elected Fellow of the Royal College of Physicians of London. Later became Vice-president.

1938 Hitler's ultimatum. Copeman's club (Athenaeum) prepares a gas proof cellar.

1939 Copeman elected Orator of the Heberden Society.

1939 Launch of the *Annals of Rheumatic Diseases*. Copeman serves on the editorial committee *ex-officio* as Medical Secretary of the Empire Rheumatism Council (ERC).

1939-45. War service. Awarded OBE.

1946 British League Against Rheumatism formed (Officers: WSC Copeman, O Savage and GH Kersley) so as to have a common rheumatology 'front' through which anyone interested in the rheumatic diseases could affiliate to the International League Against Rheumatism (ILAR) while maintaining the exclusiveness and restricted membership of the Heberden Society.

1948 First edition of Copeman's '*Textbook of the Rheumatic Diseases*'. Subsequent editions 1953, 1964,1969 (reprinted 1970). Continued under editorship of JT Scott 1978 and 1986.

1951 European League Against Rheumatism (EULAR) formed with Copeman as first President.

1954 Copeman takes over as Editor of the *Annals of Rheumatic Diseases,* continues until 1970.

1954 Copeman sets up the Heberden Library in the Royal College of Physicians and becomes the Heberden Librarian, a position he held for 16 years.

1966 Kennedy Institute opened, following negotiations by Copeman with the Kennedy's and Charing Cross Hospital.

candidature as a young rheumatologist had scientific 'added value' in that he had taken a degree in biochemistry at Cambridge. He found Copeman austere, dominating and overbearing, his questions intrusive and personal. He decided that he would not work for him. Nevertheless on parting Copeman told him to come to the Hospital of St John and Elizabeth the following morning -and he did. There he found himself subjected to a further trial by ordeal, with Copeman, so he perceived, being sarcastic and supercilious. Glyn was finally asked to discuss the case of a patient with back pain. Fortunately, a sympathetic nun-nurse had whispered to him that it was a haemangioma of the third lumbar vertebra. After that all was plain sailing. He came to like and respect Copeman and in return was treated with respect.

Copeman had the ability and personality to raise money for the Empire (*later Arthritis and -)* Rheumatism Council (ARC). Dr Tom Scott recalls that Copeman was being given a cheque by a businessman. Standing over the donor as the cheque was being written and seeing the sum, Copeman exclaimed 'Oh, but I was expecting considerably more than that!' The businessman duly added another '0' to the figure!

Moreover Copeman appreciated the need to do favours for the rich or politically powerful in the expectation of a substantial *quid pro quo* for the charity. The boss of the Joe Lyons' catering empire was Glyn's uncle who had a daughter with leukaemia. Sir Lionel Whitby had said that he could do nothing for her, but added that 'this new drug from America, cortisone, might do some good'. At the time John Glyn had a stock of cortisone in his domestic refrigerator, to be used in the UK Cortisone/Aspirin trial in rheumatoid arthritis. His uncle telephoned and said 'I want it'. Glyn refused, but referred him to Copeman. Copeman immediately authorised the release of the cortisone. Within three days it had been replaced, despite Customs' restrictions on its importation. (It did not, of course, influence the outcome. She died.) In 1960, in preparation for a conference that Copeman was to chair, a literature search for early references to the medical use of salicylates happened to find a paper by Wm. Heberden on purpura in children, clearly a forerunner of the descriptions by Henoch and Schönlein to whom posterity has given the credit. Copeman was pleased to be told of another link between Heberden and rheumatology, and of the interest 'in our eponymous hero'.

Another anecdote: (John Glyn again). Copeman found himself sitting at a dinner next to the Prosector of the London Zoo. To make conversation Copeman asked his neighbour why animals did not get osteoarthritis. "Oh but they do" the Prosector replied. Next week a box of bones from various animals with osteoarthritis was received, including the bones of a parrot that had died of gout. (This incident may be the stimulus to one of Copeman's few scientific papers, given to the Section of Comparative Medicine at the Royal Society of Medicine, describing osteoarthritis in racehorses).

Professor Norman Ashton, FRS, was an ophthalmic pathologist who discovered hyperoxic damage to the eyes of neonates. He had the idea of setting up an independent Research Institute of Ophthalmology that would serve all eye hospitals and departments. This was the model adopted by Dr Frank Dudley Hart in 1959 for a special research unit for rheumatic diseases. The original plan for it to be built in Vincent Square, London fell through but the idea was taken up by Copeman and the opportunity to realise it came in 1961, as a result of a gift by Mrs. Mathilde Kennedy, who was born a Miss Mathilde Marks, younger sister of Sir Simon Marks and heir to some of the Marks and Spencer money. She had married Terence Kennedy, idiosyncratic and a rich man in his own right and, according to opinion at that time, more interested in men than women. Mathilde, overweight and unloved, formed a strong attachment to her doctor, Dr Lankaster, who was crippled by osteoarthritis of the hips. Mathilde diverted some of the Marks charity money to fund a rheumatism research centre. With Copeman on board, the project was taken round other London teaching hospitals. In some it was viewed as an onerous benefaction and declined. It was finally accepted by the Charing Cross Hospital and was to have been incorporated into the new Charing Cross Hospital in Fulham Palace Road, but that fell through. There was enough money (about half a million pounds) to build the Institute in Bute Street, Hammersmith, adjacent to the West London Hospital. Named the Kennedy Institute, it was opened in 1966 under its own committee.

But there was insufficient money fully to endow and maintain it and it had to be subsidised by the ARC. Members of the ARC research subcommittee demurred. They took the view that money subscribed to the ARC should go into research, not into the maintenance of a building. On this occasion Copeman used his position as Chairman of the Executive of the ARC to take over the Chair of the Research Committee. Very much the senior officer in command, he denounced those professors with faint hearts who could not see the importance to rheumatology of a dedicated and independent research Institute.

As a young member of the pre-war Athenaeum, Copeman could have been classed as a benevolent medical aristocrat, who reflected the society of his day in its culture and accepted attitudes. In September 1938 he wrote of when Chamberlain returned from Godesburg with news of the impending crisis. He described the provision of gas masks, sandbags and a gas-proof room at the Athenaeum in anticipation of war. Later, when Prime Minister Neville Chamberlain was able to announce that Hitler had postponed his ultimatum, "There was very little talk of food hoarding, except for the Jews, who tried to make the shops take it all back when the danger was over." It was the sort of thing that could be said in joke then. Few realised then just what was being planned for Jewish people in Europe. And the following year when the war did begin and Copeman was drafted overseas, he wrote a poignant 4-page poem, scanned and rhymed, to his daughter 'Piggy' (Priscilla) describing his life in the tents and other events.

Copeman will be seen by history as one of the most important progenitors of modern rheumatology. There were others who shared his vision.

Dr Ernest Tertius Decimus Fletcher (1881-1961) qualified from St Bartholomew's Hospital Medical School in 1918, later joining the staff as Assistant Physician. As such he would have helped in training Dr Evelyn Hess, one of the first UK women rheumatologists, who later joined Morris Ziff's unit in Dallas and went on to be professor of Medicine. Fletcher's wartime and immediate post-war service with the army steered him towards an interest in rehabilitation and thence to the rheumatic diseases. He published one of the first textbooks of rheumatology in 1947, entitled

'Medical Disorders of the Locomotor System' that went to two editions. He was a leading figure in the Arthur Stanley Institute of the Middlesex Hospital when this evolved from the British Red Cross Society's Clinic for Rheumatism in 1948. He had been Heberden Orator in 1938 and the Heberden Society's President from 1956-7.

Professor (later Sir) Francis Fraser (1885-1979) played an important part in the new age of rheumatology. He was born in 1885 and qualified in 1910. The first Professorial Chair of Medicine at the Postgraduate School of Medicine at Hammersmith Hospital was established in 1934 with Sir Francis, until then Professor of Medicine at St Bartholomew's hospital, the first holder. Prof. Bywaters has written: "Francis Fraser at Hammersmith in 1936 encouraged the first rheumatologist there, Geoffrey Jennings[1], to write an article on 'Aspirin in Gout'- a break through! I succeeded him and took on Fraser's rheumatoid arthritis patients".

After the war Fraser became Director of the British Postgraduate Medical Federation, where he was an influential supporter of the then newly emerging specialty of rheumatology. His contribution was recognised when he was made an Honorary Member of the Heberden Society.

Lord Horder (1871-1955) (Fig 1.3) was an outstanding physician of his time and could be taken as the 'Father Figure' of a number of twentieth-century developments in Medicine. He seems to have inherited the genes for intelligence, amiability and practicality in good measure. Born in 1871, a draper's son and a scholarship boy, he won prizes at his medical school (Ss. Bartholomew's) from which he qualified in 1900. After junior jobs and service in the First World War he joined the staff of St Bartholomew's and became a full physician in 1921.

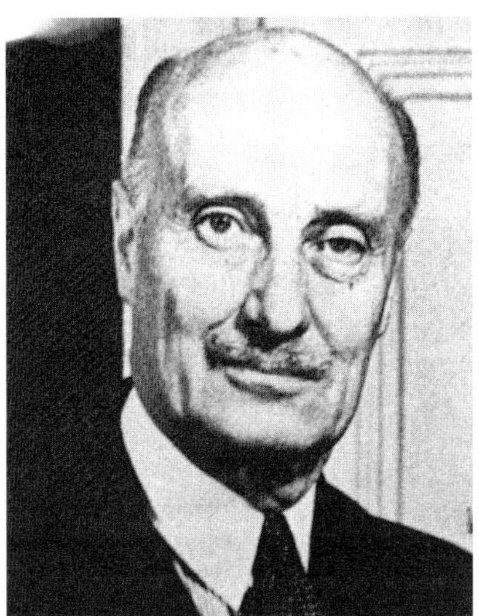

Figure 1.2 Dr WSC Copeman

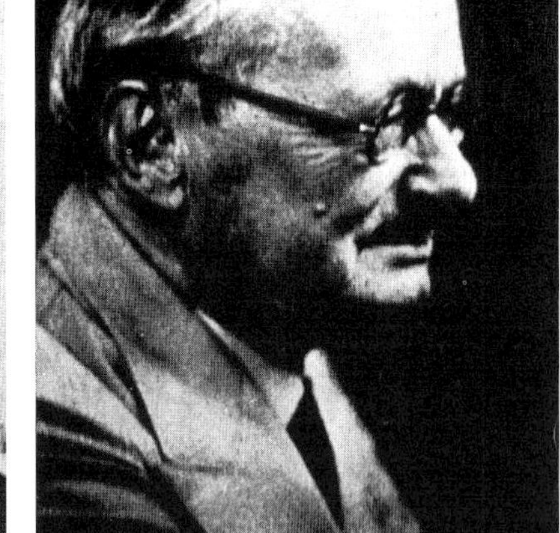

Figure 1.3 Lord Horder

1 Rheumatology was not Jennings' prime interest. During the war Jennings transferred as general physician to the Redhill Hospital in Edgeware, later known as the Edgeware General Hospital. At that point his scientific output virtually ceased.

He used to allow school boys and girls to wander through the grounds of his house in Steep, near Petersfield. Horder once gave a lecture (lucidly) on obscurantism. His theme was the way in which professionals and politicians hide what they want to convey behind invented verbiage, long words and circumlocutions, a lesson still needed today when every medical journal and computer manual has its own private vocabulary of abbreviations, acronyms and neologisms.

It is unclear whether Horder or Copeman first had the idea of pursuing the concept of rheumatology as a separate specialty of medicine, to be lifted out of its low status in the medical hierarchy in the between war years as a province of physical medicine. Copeman began to work with Horder in his middle 20s. He was nearly 30 years Horder's junior. Horder was already rich and famous and physician to the Prince of Wales. Copeman must have done most of the leg-work and letter writing which led to the meetings that were to set up the National Association for Combating Rheumatism in 1928. The Association was a precursor of the Empire Rheumatism Council (ERC).

Dr George Kersley who was taught by Horder at St Bartholomew's Hospital clearly hero–worshipped Horder and positioned himself in a similar way, supporting the ERC, the Heberden Society, the British Association for Physical Medicine and the British Rheumatism Association with equal favour. Kersley contrasted Horder with Sir Francis Fraser. Fraser was deductive and diagnosed by exclusion while Horder was inductive and intuitive. According to Kersley (Kersley and Glyn, 1991) Horder 'was never wrong'.

Horder was Chairman of the Empire Rheumatism Council from 1936 to 1953. It was Horder who decided that the first Scientific Advisory Committee was too cumbersome and reduced the number from 34 to 10, thereby excluding Francis Bach. It seems unlikely that he would have done this without first consulting Copeman.

Horder was catholic in his patronage. He presided over a large number of medical societies as well as being active in rheumatology. He was President of the Heberden Society in 1953 and first President of the British Association for Physical Medicine, serving from 1943 to the year of his death in 1955. He allowed his name to be attached to the Horder Centres for Arthritics and the organisation of Horder Helpers started by Miss Cecilia Bochenek that at one time were raising more money than the Empire Rheumatism Council. The only organisation in which he does not seem to have taken a leading position was the British Rheumatism Association (later renamed Arthritis Care). Unlike Copeman, he did not see rheumatology and physical medicine as adversaries.

George Kersley (1906-1992) was born and died in the city of Bath and lived there all his life apart from the years spent in training and his war service in the Middle East. When he retired from medicine he was elected Mayor of Bath. He so identified himself with the city of Bath that the affectionate joke was that it was George Kersley who was the real 'George' of Georgian Bath. He had qualified in Cambridge and St Bartholomew's, soon gained his MRCP and won a prize for his MD thesis. Lord Horder encouraged him to practice rheumatology although this was not highly rated by the medical profession at the time. In 1934 he was appointed to do general medicine (which he later gave up) in the Royal United Hospital in Bath plus rheumatology at the

Royal Mineral Water Hospital, as it was then named. He spearheaded the change of name to the Royal National Hospital for Rheumatic Diseases in 1936. By 1939 he had collected funds and permission to rebuild the hospital on a larger site but the war intervened and the money was sequestrated. He was a founder member in 1939 of the Empire Rheumatism Council [Figure 1.4] and in that role he found himself bridging the growing gap between Copeman and Francis Bach. Like his mentor Lord Horder, Kersley supported both rheumatology and physical medicine. He played several parts in the international scene in rheumatology. To quote his obituary by Dr. John Cosh: 'Among the many positions he held at various times were President of the European League against Rheumatism, Vice-President of the International League, President of the Heberden Society, founder member of the British Association for Physical Medicine and Deputy-Lieutenant for the County of Somerset.'

The city of Bath and the Royal National Hospital for Rheumatic Diseases were damaged in the Baedecker raids in 1942. Temporary repairs were made. At the advent of the National Health Service in 1948 there were some newly in authority in Bath who decided to close the hospital rather than restore it. They wished to incorporate it as a department of the Royal United Hospital. Kersley resisted this, successfully taking his case to the House of Lords and raising further money for the restoration and modernisation.

His experience on the Empire Rheumatism Council's Scientific Advisory Committee had convinced him of the necessity for research into rheumatoid arthritis. In 1948 he set up the Rheumatism Research Unit for the South West and Oxford Regions, to which the Oliver Bird Fund contributed the salary of Dr M. Desmarais. The Unit was later taken over by the Medical Research Council. Kersley saw to it that in 1965, when the Hospital was reopened after successful refurbishment, it would have new penthouse laboratories for clinical research. These were opened by Princess Marina of Kent.

Kersley was often involved in controversy but he was without malice. He advised that however forcefully one had to defend one's position in committee, 'always invite your adversary round for a drink afterwards' to talk informally and in this way he managed to avoid the build-up of animosities which sometimes plague hospital life.

Francis (Frank) Dudley Hart, (b. 1909) qualified at Edinburgh in 1933. At the outbreak of the war he was Medical Registrar and Emergency Medical Service Physician at the Westminster Hospital, working with two surgeons and a surgical Registrar. They had been left behind to run the hospital as a casualty clearing station in anticipation of London being bombed. The patients, teaching staff and most of the medical students had been evacuated to sector hospitals outside London. Later he served as Medical Specialist and Officer in charge of a medical division of the Royal Army Medical Corps. He wrote early papers on ankylosing spondylitis arising out of his experience of the rheumatic problems of wartime recruits, firmly differentiating this disease from other forms of chronic inflammatory arthritis. He was appointed to the staff of the Westminster Hospital in 1947, doing general medicine, when a senior colleague General Stott, who was interested in rheumatology, on returning from the Army told Hart to set up a rheumatism unit, the first in a London teaching hospital.

In 1952 the Royal College of Physicians moved from Trafalgar Square to Regent's Park. Hart, as Chairman of the College's Committee on Rheumatology, helped push through the recognition of Rheumatology as a separate specialty of Medicine.

In the course of a long life Hart has written many research papers, reviews and contributions to books. As early as 1939 he published in the first volume of the *Annals of Rheumatic Diseases* a study on the production of subcutaneous nodules in rheumatic fever. (Hart, 1939) The importance of the study scientifically was that it did *not* confirm the assertion that nodules could be experimentally produced by regularly rubbing elbow skin on the sheets. The importance of the study professionally was that it established his interest in the field.

Hart has also been an accomplished publicist for the specialty. An article on 'The Long Pain' based on the difficulty rheumatoid arthritis sufferers have in getting a full night's undisturbed sleep is still remembered. He has through the columns of the Arthritis and Rheumatism Council's news-sheet explained to the lay readership the many different rheumatic diseases and their problems. He did an early survey of complementary medicine. Of 140 rheumatism patients approached, 111 replied. Of those who had tried various forms of complementary medicine 40% felt they were helped by faith healing, 50% by acupuncture and 80% by osteopathy or manipulation.

He was one of the first Secretaries of the Heberden Society and from 1957 to 1972 served as its Honorary Treasurer. Hart and the Honorary Librarian (Copeman) were the only members of the Heberden Executive that did not have a fixed term of office, so they had an avuncular role that ensured the continuity of policy of the Society. He was also a long-term member of the committees of the Arthritis and Rheumatism Council, where his role was somewhat similar, maintaining due balance between the claims of basic and clinical research and restraining the endless avidity of laboratory scientists for more funds.

In his 91st year he remains very active. In Japan he would not only be a 'Father Figure' but might be classed as a 'Living National Monument'.

Oswald Arthur Savage (1907-1995)(Fig 1.4.) qualified from St Bartholomew's Hospital in 1932. He met Copeman during war service and Copeman put him in charge of the Medical Division of the 65th General Hospital. Savage had been a Medical Registrar at St Stephen's Hospital and written a paper on the oxygen and carbon dioxide tensions in the knee joint in normal and pathological conditions. Later with Francis Bach he described three patients who had had splenectomy for Felty's Syndrome, with 'remarkable improvement in two of them' (Bach and Savage, 1940)

After his war service, for which he was awarded the OBE, Copeman made him Honorary Medical Secretary of the Empire Rheumatism Council (later renamed Arthritis and Rheumatism Council) a job in which he remained for 22 years. Copeman arranged for him to be appointed to the Middlesex Hospital with sessions in rheumatic diseases at the then West London Hospital. He helped Copeman as assistant editor of the 'Annals of Rheumatic Diseases'; the word being that Savage did most of the work.

The author was nominated by Savage as second Assistant Secretary of the European League against Rheumatism (EULAR) in 1964, a job held for fourteen years,

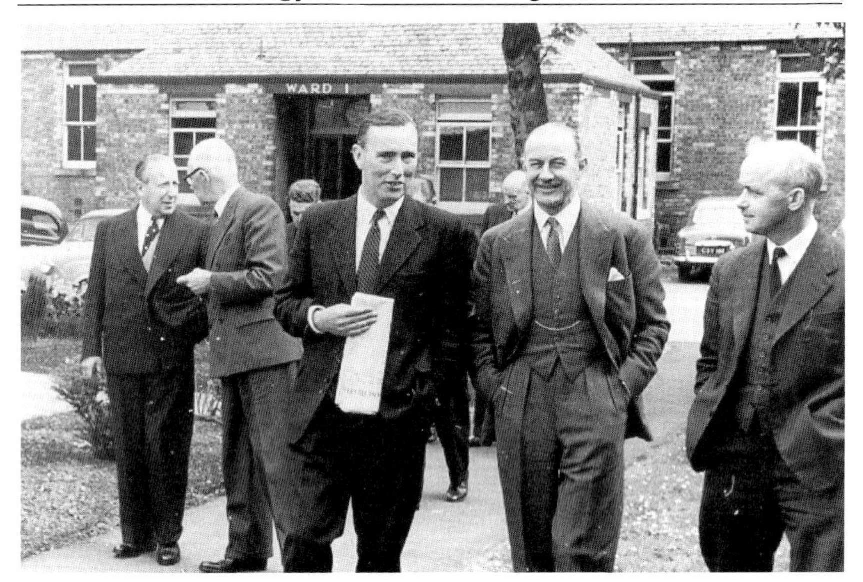

Figure 1.4. Meeting of the Heberden Society at the Northern General Hospital, Edinburgh in 1955. From the left: *Francis Bach, Sir Stanley Davidson, Alan Hill (*background), *George Fearnley, Will Copeman* (background), *Oswald Savage, Harry West.*

with promotion to first Assistant then Secretary-General as the seniors died in office. (Not wishing to follow them it was decided to change the Constitution of the League so as to ensure no more than a 4-year term of office for its office-holders!)

Savage's research was mainly on the effects of adrenocorticotrophic hormone (ACTH) and cortisone in the rheumatic diseases. He was an advocate of the patient administering her own ACTH. When he retired and was no longer under the shadow of Copeman he seems to have wanted to get away from it all and to develop his own personality. He moved with his wife Kitty to the sun and wine of the good life in the South of France in 1969, where he had his own vineyard. (Contractors picked the grapes and made the wine, returning it to him in bottles. He admitted later that it did not save any money but it was nice to have.) He became an accomplished painter and 'had an oil landscape hung in the Royal Academy in 1982" (Moll)

He was seen as a quiet sort of man, friendly, efficient, a 'good civil servant', remembered with affection by those who worked with him and someone who was always accessible to those who served on the ARC Committees.

Francis Bach was amongst the 33 members of the Scientific Advisory Committee of the Empire Rheumatism Council in 1936 (Fig 1.5.) This committee effectively ran the Council. To be on it was a privilege. But it was unmanageable and when Lord Horder demoted some members including Bach to minor subcommittees, Bach seems to have taken umbrage. A further episode occurred about 1946. Oswald Savage had been Bach's registrar at St Stephen's Hospital before the war, working for both Bach and Philip Ellman. Ellman was a respiratory physician in one hospital in

London, and a rheumatologist in St Stephen's. He is important to the history of rheumatology because in this dual role he made original observations on the rheumatoid lung, and later coined the term 'rheumatoid disease' to emphasise that rheumatoid arthritis was a multi-system disorder. Savage joined up early in the War and served overseas, Bach remained at home, a member of the Emergency Medical Service. After the war Bach failed to reinstate Savage as might have been expected. Certainly Bach took no further part in the activities of the ERC, or ARC as it later became.

The British Rheumatism Association was set up in 1947 largely as a continuation of the Charterhouse Clinics under Dr Warren Crowe but soon came to be identified with Bach (the abbreviation 'BRA' was joked about as 'Bach's Rheumatism Association). The founders intended it to provide help, education and welfare services such as sheltered accommodation, holiday homes and local support groups for arthritis sufferers. Whereas the ARC was purely educational and scientific and had no public membership, membership of the BRA was open to individual sufferers and those who cared for them. Copeman saw this as possible competition, including for funds. A *modus vivendi* evolved in which the ARC did not recruit a formal membership and the BRA did not raise funds for research. However there was some overlap in, for example the provision of explanatory booklets about the various rheumatic diseases. Moreover the BRA did put a cautious toe in the research pool when it funded a study by Drs April Kay and Francis Bach on the impaired fertility of women before they developed rheumatoid arthritis. Bach was once asked 'why couldn't the ARC and the BRA join up?' He said it would never happen because the paid directors of these organizations had too much vested interest in remaining separate. Perhaps they still do.

Francis Bach had been a Registrar at Peto Place before the war and had contributed to a survey of beds available to rheumatic fever sufferers in London. That survey was published in the first issue of the *Annals of Rheumatic Diseases* (Bach et al, 1939). With Freedman he published one of the first studies of mepacrine in rheumatoid arthritis (Freedman and Bach, 1952). He wrote one of the early (1955) textbooks of Physical Medicine, (it included rheumatology) that was quite well received although one reviewer, (Bywaters) stigmatized two of the illustrations as 'crossword puzzles without clues'. Bach recommended splenectomy for Felty's syndrome, advice that has on the right occasion been dramatically successful. Others have stressed the failures and recurrences after splenectomy but the modern treatment with granulocyte colony stimulating factor also has its problems and failures. (Stanworth et al.,1998)

Dr Douglas Woolf, who had followed Bach as Registrar to the Red Cross Clinic in Peto Place and who later became a trustee of the British Rheumatism Association recalled that the work of seeing the patients at Peto Place was left largely to the Registrar with little supervision. The staff members would come, smoke, take tea and discuss.

Two other persons need to be noticed in this section. It is a tenable proposition that they did more for rheumatic disease sufferers than any rheumatologist. One was Sir John Charnley for his single-minded development of the total hip replacement arthroplasty bonded to bone by an adhesive developed from dental cement. Charnley had been working on this at the Manchester Royal Infirmary in the 1950s,

MEMBERS OF THE SCIENTIFIC ADVISORY
COMMITTEE OF THE EMPIRE RHEUMATISM COUNCIL

MERVYN H. GORDON, C.M.G., C.B.E., F.R.S., D.M. (*Chairman*).

F. J. BACH, D.M.
LADY RUTH BALFOUR, M.B., M.R.C.S., L.R.C.P.
C. W. BUCKLEY, M.D., F.R.C.P.
E. T. CONYBEARE, M.D., F.R.C.P.
PROFESSOR L. S. P. DAVIDSON, M.D., F.R.C.P.E., F.R.S.E.
PROFESSOR E. C. DODDS, M.V.O., M.D., F.R.C.P.
JAMES FENTON, C.B.E., M.D., M.R.C.P.
A. G. TIMBRELL FISHER, M.C., F.R.C.S.
R. F. FOX, M.D., F.R.C.P.
PROFESSOR F. R. FRASER, M.D., F.R.C.P.
SIR HENRY GAUVAIN, M.A., M.D., F.R.C.S.
TOM HARE, M.D., M.R.C.V.S.
PROFESSOR SIR LEONARD HILL, F.R.S., LL.D., M.B.
G. HOLMES, M.B.
G. D. KERSLEY, M.D., M.R.C.P.
PROFESSOR R. J. S. MCDOWALL, M.D., D.SC., F.R.C.P.E.
PROFESSOR T. J. MACKIE, M.D., M.R.C.P.
PROFESSOR W. M. MITCHELL, F.R.C.V.S.
J. LEWIN PAYNE, O.B.E., M.R.C.S., L.R.C.P., L.D.S.
PROFESSOR C. BRUCE PERRY, M.D., F.R.C.P.
E. P. POULTON, D.M., F.R.C.P.
M. B. RAY, D.S.O., M.D., M.R.C.P.
PROFESSOR W. T. RITCHIE, O.B.E., F.R.C.P.E.
SIR HUMPHRY ROLLESTON, BT., G.C.V.O., K.C.B., M.D., F.R.C.P.
W. S. TEGNER, M.R.C.P.
E. C. WARNER, M.D., F.R.C.P.
PROFESSOR G. W. WATSON, M.D., F.R.C.P.
LIONEL WHITBY, C.V.O., M.D., F.R.C.P.
SIR WILLIAM WILLCOX, K.C.I.E., C.B., C.M.G., M.D., F.R.C.P.
SIR ROBERT STANTON WOODS, M.D., F.R.C.P.

LORD HORDER, G.C.V.O., M.D., F.R.C.P., *Chairman*, and
W. S. C. COPEMAN, M.D., F.R.C.P.Lond., *Medical Secretary*
of the Council are *ex officio* members.

Fig 1.5. Members of the Scientific Advisory Committee of the Red Cross Clinic for Rheumatism. (From the Clinic's Annual Report for 1946).

culminating in him being given permission to set up a dedicated hip unit at the Wrightington Hospital in 1958.

The other was Sir Ernst Chain who gave the world penicillin. He also discovered penicillamine, although the usefulness of penicillamine in rheumatoid arthritis would not become apparent for more than twenty years. To quote John Moll (1987) on Chain:

'The work of Chain and colleagues led to the virtual elimination of infective arthritis caused by penicillin-sensitive organisms (gonococci, streptococci, treponemata and other organisms). The discovery also led to the saving of rheumatic children and prevented much chronic heart disease.'

And let Aneurin Bevan not be forgotten. He was the father of the National Health Service, which bestowed a great privilege on those who dealt with patients who had chronic diseases that interfered with the capacity to earn money. Private doctors needed to charge for their services. Under the NHS one could give with one hand without having to take with the other.

The Setting in 1948

Undergraduates had been taught rheumatology during the war in terms of eponymous heroes: Hippocrates for his aphorisms on gout; Sydenham's chorea; Charcot's joints; Clutton's joints, Dupuytren's contracture; Heberden's nodes; Baker's cysts; Garrod for his insights into uric acid and gout; Still for Still's Disease.

H Reiter, AR Felty, and H Sjögren and their syndromes did not feature at the time. This 'sound-bite' teaching was mirrored on the wards. Asked about rheumatoid arthritis the student was expected to answer 'ulnar deviation of the fingers', ankylosing spondylitis went with 'bamboo spine' and rheumatic fever with red hair[2] and heart murmurs.

To be fair to the deficiencies of teaching, it was wartime. Younger staff had been recruited to the Services. Those who remained were doctors recalled from retirement or exempted on health or essential services grounds. The authorities, expecting many casualties from bombs on the metropolis and bigger cities, evacuated civilian patients to a halo of district sector hospitals to free beds in the cities. Pre-clinical and first year clinical students went with them. Frank Dudley Hart, then a medical registrar, recalls that Westminster Hospital was emptied of normal services and was left to him and other relatively junior doctors to run as a casualty reception and clearing station. Guy's preclinical and clinical students were moved to Kent, later to be underneath the action and bombs during the Battle of Britain. Subsequently the more experienced students were transferred back to the mother hospital in time to experience the disruption caused by the flying bombs and V2 rockets. What one learnt centred on trauma and death, not rheumatology.

In 1945, when the war ended, some senior students from Guy's went to Belsen to witness the horrors and tend the survivors of the concentration camps. Armed services doctors were gradually 'de-mobbed' and given money for retraining, leading in some to postgraduate degrees. That achieved, specialisation, research and promotion up the job ladder to consultant status beckoned, cardiology being for many a favourite choice. The word research was glamorous, the reality often humdrum but the possibilities were vastly increased by the advent of the National Health Service which from its inception held medical research to be amongst its objects. All hospital treatment was free at the time of need, any patient could go into any hospital, snobbish distinction between the up-market ex-voluntary hospitals and the down-market ex-poor law or local authority hospitals disappeared, at least in theory. There was money for reconstruction and some for research. The Medical Research Council and the large charitable medical foundations became active again. Doctors, not administrators, controlled the hospitals. It was a time of energy, enthusiasm and change, characterised by the Festival of Britain in 1951.

Before, during and immediately after the war there were few places in London where women could train in medicine. The main school for them was at the Royal Free Hospital in Gray's Inn Road, which did not admit men students. A limited

4 One consultant who believed strongly in the association with hair colour, but who had observed exceptions, subdivided red hair into goldilocks, copperknob, carrots and ginger and said that only 'carrots'held the predisposition. As a young houseman he had observed carrot-coloured hair in a 5-year old with rheumatic

number of places were reserved for women at King's College, St George's, University College, the Middlesex and West London Hospitals. From 1948 to 1970 few women became hospital consultants and even fewer went into rheumatology. Early exceptions were Dr Barbara Ansell at Taplow and Northwick Park and Dr Mary Carter at St Mary's. Drs Jean Colston, Mary Corbett and Professor Ann Chamberlain came from departments originally labelled Physical Medicine. By 1960 all medical schools admitted men and women on an equal basis but in 1997 of 371 UK Consultant Rheumatologists less than 1 in 10 were women. (British Society for Rheumatology, Handbook 1997).

The greatest change in the five years after the war was in the battle against the infectious diseases. Sulphanilamide had been identified as the active part of the antibiotic dye Prontosil before the war but more effective derivatives had emerged. Alexander Fleming had in 1929 published his observation that the mould *Penicillium* secreted a substance that killed staphylococci in vitro, but he failed to try it in vivo. There the matter had rested until Ernst Chain working with Howard Florey in Oxford in 1942 rediscovered Fleming's paper and set about analysing the active principle.

Intensive collaborative work between the USA and the UK discovered more productive strains of the mould. Alterations to the growth medium together with X-ray and ultraviolet irradiation of the spores had raised the yield of penicillin 1000-fold compared to that of Fleming's original strain. At first supplies were reserved for the war wounded but by 1947 were widely available to the civil population. A few Gram-negative and all Gram-positive bacteria except the tubercle bacillus were susceptible. Antibiotic resistance had not yet emerged. Gonorrhoeal, streptococcal, staphylococcal and pneumococcal forms of septic arthritis suddenly became easily treatable. Streptomycin was introduced in 1948, and for the first time one saw rapid recovery in young adults suffering from tuberculous arthritis and spinal disease. The days of artificial pneumothorax, thoracoplasties and phrenic nerve crushes to collapse cavities in the lung were numbered, as were the tuberculosis hospitals themselves, some of which, like Black Notley and Leasoe in England and Baird Street in Glasgow, were later to be taken over for rheumatic diseases.The introduction of streptomycin had another important result. Supplies were at first limited. Under the guidance of Austin (Tony) Bradford Hill as statistician and of Drs Guy Scadding and John Crofton at the Brompton Hospital and others the opportunity was taken to conduct a controlled trial comparing treated with untreated tuberculous patients. This proved the value of streptomycin beyond all doubt. So started the Bradford Hill revolution in evidence-based therapeutics that was to have enormous consequences for the verification of efficacy of new treatments for the rheumatic diseases.

Post-streptococcal rheumatic fever and chorea were to take a little longer to conquer. The Group A, β-haemolytic streptocooccus had increased in virulence with the privations and herding together of children and young recruits during the war but rheumatic fever had been waning in seriousness even before the use of antibiotics. Ten

Footnote 2 Contd. fever, later in a child with St. Vitus' Dance, then when he became a registrar he saw a young women with rheumatic heart disease and mitral stenosis. Later still, as a consultant he looked after a woman in atrial fibrillation and heart failure. All had this striking coloured hair. What he hadn't registered was that they were all the same person.

years later, rheumatic fever, once a disease affecting 80,000 children in the UK and killing many, was to become so rare that most doctors then recruited to rheumatology would never see it.

1948 was an *annus mirabilis* for rheumatology in the United Kingdom. The antibiotics and other potent drugs became available and there were new opportunities offered by the National Health Service. In the USA Rose rediscovered the rheumatoid factor previously described by Waaler but overlooked during the war and Hargraves discovered the Lupus Cell phenomenon. Phenylbutazone, the first powerful non-steroidal anti-inflammatory drug after aspirin, was coming into use as co-therapy with amidopyrine in the Geigy preparation called Irgapyrine. In 1952, phenylbutazone was reported by Currie (1952) to be active in its own right.

But more spectacular was the news from across the Atlantic of the introduction of cortisone and corticotrophin, then called adrenocorticotrophic hormone (ACTH). Important, too, was the effect on raising the estimation of rheumatology amongst medical colleagues as an integral part of general internal medicine. Before 1948 it could be said that: 'rheumatology is like dermatology, your patients never die and they never get you out of bed at night'. Corticosteroids changed that. Their misuse or sudden withdrawal could provoke a life-threatening emergency. Special blue 'Steroid identity cards' were issued so that patients taken to hospital after a collapse or accident could carry with them the details of the corticosteroid and dose they had been taking.

Chapter 2.
Academic Development in the Second Half of the 20th Century

The first three academic Chairs of rheumatology were established at Manchester, London, and Edinburgh with JH Kellgren, EGL Bywaters, and JJR Duthie respectively as professors. The money to endow the chairs and support the research did not come from governmental or University Grants Commission sources, but from two major charitable funding bodies, the Oliver Bird Fund of the Nuffield Foundation and the Arthritis and Rheumatism Council.

The three men were born and qualified in Medicine within a few months of each other. The academic legacies they have left differ. Bywaters with his prior training on pathology and his double base at Hammersmith and Taplow will be remembered for conducting superb observational studies on rheumatic diseases in children and adults, Kellgren will be remembered for his pioneering studies on the epidemiology of rheumatic diseases and Duthie for the large number of highly competent rheumatolgists he trained as well as his early studies on industrial rheumatic diseases.

London. EGL Bywaters and the Postgraduate Medical School at Hammersmith Hospital

Eric Bywaters (fig 2.1) was born in 1910. The family business, which had for five generations been the building of hotels and apartments in the UK and Europe, was called 'Aquis Property Company,' aquis being the Latin for 'by waters'. He had a happy and successful undergraduate career, graduating from the Middlesex Hospital in 1933 with a gold medal and Honours in pathology. His post-registration house appointments were followed by appointment as assistant clinical pathologist to the Bland Sutton Institute at the hospital. While working there and doing biochemical research on cartilage with Sir Charles Dodds at the Courtauld Institute he was visited by

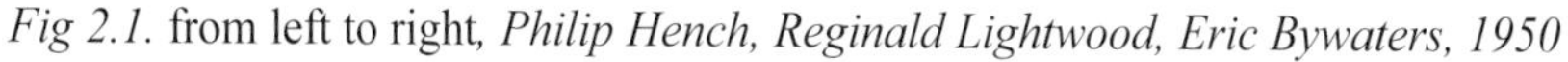

Fig 2.1. from left to right, *Philip Hench, Reginald Lightwood, Eric Bywaters, 1950*

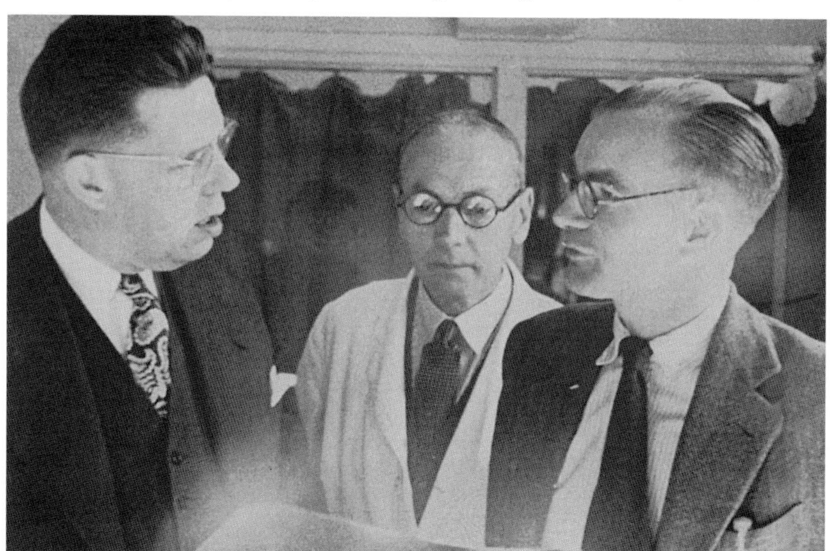

Dr Walter Bauer who offered him a Fellowship at the Massachusetts General Hospital (MGH), promising him large numbers of calf joints for study. Supplemented by a Rockerfeller travelling fellowship, he and his wife Betty worked in Boston for two years. His main clinical research interest there was lupus erythematosus. Betty did the follow-ups. Supported by a Beit Memorial Fellowship, he came back to Hammersmith Hospital in 1939 which he later recalled as "the only place then the UK equal of the MGH". Later he was appointed as Consultant and Senior Lecturer in general medicine with a special interest in rheumatic diseases at the Postgraduate Medical School at Hammersmith Hospital. The word 'rheumatologist' had at that time hardly been invented.

He had time to assemble a series of patients with rheumatoid arthritis treated along conventional lines before 1940 when hostilities really began. His research was redirected to wound shock and the crush syndrome in industrial injuries and bomb victims. In 1944 he took over the Medical Research Council Shock Research Unit in Newcastle under Ronald Grant when the latter moved to the battle areas. Bywaters with Erasmus Barlow and Jean Stead continued the work on the crush syndrome in industrial accidents and in bomb victims whose limbs had been trapped and crushed by falling masonry and who, after release by the rescue services, developed anuria and renal failure. The cause, he found, was ischaemic lysis of muscle cells that on reperfusion released myoglobin into the bloodstream and blocked the tubules in the kidneys. Bywaters used animal models to show that alkaline fluids by mouth or intravenously could prevent renal damage and the patient kept alive until the blocked renal tubules could heal. Assisted by Drs Graham Bull and Jo Joekes he installed the Kolf artificial kidney, working on it from 1945-6

Fig 2.2. Hammersmith Hospital in 1950. From a lithography by Albany Wiseman

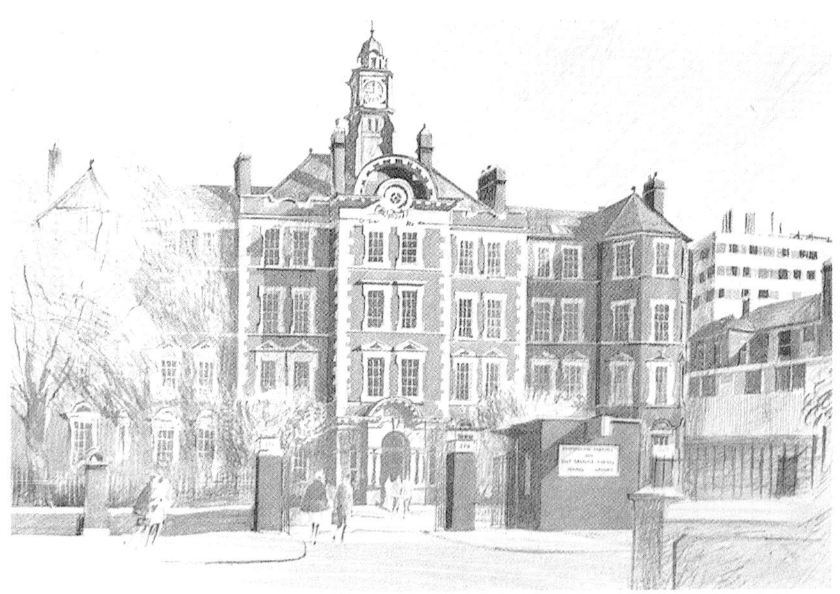

In 1947 young doctors returning from service overseas and seeking postgraduate training were employed as house officers at the Hammersmith Hospital (Fig 2.2) at a salary of £11 per month plus keep. The place was humming with research activity. There was a near 100 percent autopsy rate and a climate of calling into consultation any and every member of the staff who might conceivably have an interest in a patient's disease.

Bywaters was one of many on the staff at the time who were to make notable contributions to Medicine. By 1948 he had taken on an even more fulfilling role. In 1947 he had been appointed Director of the Special Unit for Juvenile Rheumatism at the Canadian Red Cross Memorial Hospital at Taplow. (Paediatric rheumatology will be considered further in chapter 7). This was theoretically a separate job but from Bywaters' standpoint the Taplow and Hammersmith work were totally integrated. Those he trained or who came to him on Fellowships were considered to be part of both hospitals. Dr Richard Watts followed by Dr George Fearnley (Fig 1.4.) were his full time consultant colleagues. He was also helped by a research Registrar, Dr Ellis Dresner. Dresner was funded by the Nuffield Foundation to continue the follow-up of the series of rheumatoid arthritis patients who had been kept on a register since 1939.

That survey led to an accumulation of clinical and pathological data that has been the basis of numerous studies of the natural history of rheumatoid arthritis and the causes of death in that disease. It also documented recovery from rheumatoid arthritis. (Tracing some of the original patients required the use of a detective agency. One man was found who was perfectly well, apart from being 20 years older and having some residual limitation of wrist movement.)

Ready access to specimens and histological material through the pathology department and post mortem room (Professors Dible, Harrison and Doniach) together with Bywaters' own earlier training in pathology led to studies of the morbid anatomy of the rheumatic diseases. The most notable were work on lung and heart disease in rheumatoid arthritis and other connective tissue diseases. Bywaters also studied nodules, bursae and tendon lesions. In 1958 he was appointed ARC Professor of Rheumatology and in 1962 received the Gairdner Award.

In 1957 the author joined the team (Fig 2.3) after Fearnley had moved to Gloucester. It seemed important to emphasise the 'General Medicine' part of the job and a programme of 'near-patient' research was started on topics that would not look too narrowly rheumatological on a *Curriculum Vitae* and publication list. With Drs Philip Wood and Tom Scott the recently developed ^{51}chromium red cell labelling technique was used to study fecal blood loss caused by aspirin and other non-steroidal anti-inflammatory agents. This culminated in an International Symposium on Salicylates. The team published studies on gout, hyperuricaemia, hyperparathyroidism, acromegaly, Forestier's disease and on digital vasculitis in rheumatoid arthritis. John Webb and Howard Duncan from Australia co-authored papers on the joint and muscle problems of haemophilia sufferers and on a unique family suffering from hyperuricaemic nephropathy respectively.

Rheumatology was accepted by most of the consultant staff at Hammersmith to be at the heart of general medicine and far removed from traditional

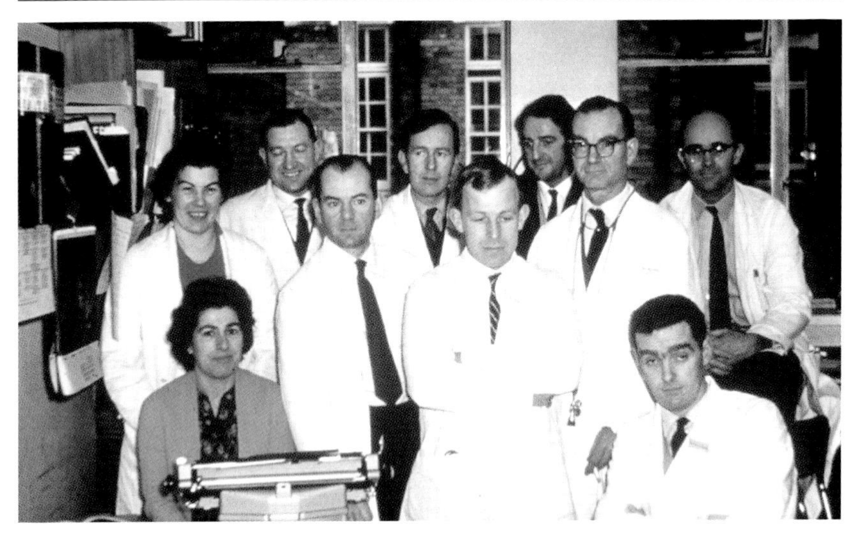

Fig 2.3. The team at Hammersmith in 1959. Sitting left, *Beryl Howard, Secretary,* Standing from left, *Barbara Ansell, Walter Boyd, Allan Dixon, Philip Wood, John Jefferis, Dick Wigley, Eric Bywaters, Tom Scott.* Sitting right, *Dermott Hourihane.*

physical medicine and spa treatment. The first controlled trial in physiotherapy with participation of the Physiotherapy department under Miss Hamilton found that the outcome of infra-red therapy with the machine switched off could not be distinguished from treatment with the machine switched on.

That systemic lupus and rheumatoid arthritis were multisystem diseases was very important for the recognition of rheumatology as a medical speciality in its own right. Not all agreed. Professor Sheila Sherlock once said that rheumatologists should be like dermatologists and not take part in general medical admissions. Some years later, when work on intra-articular pressure was presented to the Medical Research Society she complimented the presenters and said it was nice to see 'some science in Physical Medicine'. They smiled.

Whether the future of rheumatology is best served by 'pure ' rheumatologists or by those who retain an up to date competence in general medicine has long been under discussion, the tide flowing mostly in favour of rheumatology without a general medical commitment. Germane to this issue was a study of 100 consecutive emergency admissions to a general medical ward in 1981. Forty three had an associated rheumatological problem, which in 32 was a source of complaint and in 19 had either caused the admission, contributed to it or modified arrangements for treatment, nursing, rehabilitation or discharge.

There was never a problem with paediatric surgical rheumatology at Hammersmith as children could always be transferred to Taplow. However, surgical rheumatology in adults was a rather different matter. The orthopaedic contribution to rheumatology had been the subject of a discussion between the British Orthopaedic Association and the Empire *(later Arthritis and-)* Rheumatism Council as early as 1942, but little progress had been made. There had been a number of attempts to design hip arthroplasties before 1939 but their development and evaluation were interrupted as orthopaedic surgeons were occupied with war casualties at home and abroad. After the war orthopaedic surgeons rather than general surgeons were the people who looked after fractures and the trauma associated with the increasing numbers of cars on the roads. The pre-war orthopaedic surgery arising from tuberculosis, rickets and poliomyelitis had all but disappeared but was more than compensated for by the increase in consultations for non-operative conditions such as back pain and shoulder lesions. Expertise in dealing with the mechanical deformities of rheumatoid arthritis and osteoarthritis was slow to develop. Until the 1960s the McMurray osteotomy was the operation favoured by most surgeons for the treatment of osteoarthritis of the hip. Charnley and McKee had devised effective hip replacements in the 1950s but it took some time to realise that the elderly and the rheumatoid arthritic were among the best subjects for hip replacement as they would not be putting their prostheses to excessive use.

Mr (later Sir) Henry Osmond-Clarke joined the Scientific Co-ordinating Committee of the ARC in the 1960s and '70s and helped raise awareness of the possibilities of surgical rheumatology.

A large number of trainees and Fellows came through the Hammersmith firm, either directly or by rotation through Taplow. Hammersmith was a Mecca for young postgraduate doctors from the old Commonwealth. There was never a shortage of pairs of hands to run the clinics, undertake research or help look after the inpatients. Before he retired in 1975 Bywaters could count 349 who had come through his departments at Hammersmith or Taplow as housemen, registrars or research assistants, 99 from the United Kingdom. Most became consultants in rheumatology or immunology. Of the remainder no less than 33 were Canadian and there were substantial numbers from Australia and New Zealand, a rheumatological diaspora with world-wide significance.

It was at first policy not to train too many UK doctors as there were at the time few consultant jobs for them in the NHS establishment when they left. Early trainees who stayed in the London area in rheumatology included Eric Hamilton, (Kings College), Anthony Yates (St Thomas'), Mary Carter (St Mary's), Rodney Graham (Guy's), Barbara Ansell (Taplow), Tom Scott (Charing Cross), Harry Currey (The London), and Ian Meanock (Reading). Two others who might have become leaders in the speciality in this country were Ellis Dresner and Rodney Bluestone, both of whom emigrated to the USA.

'Hammersmith is a hospital where everyone is learning his job except the Heads of Departments and the Matron', said John McMichael, the Professor of Medicine. In 1961 the author moved from there first to the Chelsea and Kensington Rheumatism Unit that had been started by Bach and Ellman, subsequently to Bath in 1965. Dr.Lennox Holt was the successor. Holt in turn moved to Manchester and was succeeded in 1973 by Dr. Grahame Hughes. Hughes and his colleagues built up an international reputation for work on the lupus anti-cardiolipin factor. Bywaters retired in 1975 but continued in active research for nine years using the facility of the Arthritis and Rheumatism Council funded Bone and Joint Research Laboratories at the London

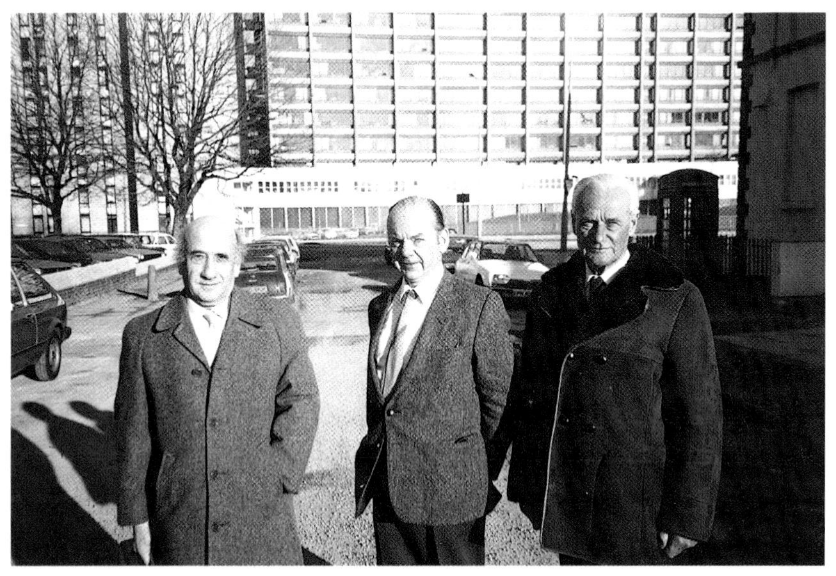

Fig 2.4. Prof John Woodrow, (Liverpool), Dr Allan Dixon and Prof. JH Kellgren (Manchester) about 1980.

Hospital. He undertook meticulous studies of the spines of those rheumatism patients who had left him their bodies for research. He 'uncovered a wealth of material left on the autopsy table and disregarded by conventional pathologists'.

Like his predecessors, Hughes left Hammersmith, (now part of the Imperial College School of Medicine). He moved to St Thomas' Hospital where he was awarded a personal Chair, supported by a substantial grant. Prof. Mark Walport, an immunologist and expert on complement and lupus took his place.

The contribution of the Hammersmith unit from 1939, aided from the earliest times by the Arthritis and Rheumatism Council, the Medical Research Council, the Wellcome Trust, the Nuffield Foundation and other funding agencies, was a major link between the speciality and general internal medicine.

Manchester. Jonas Henrick Kellgren and The Centre for Research into Chronic Rheumatic Diseases.

Jonas Henrik Kellgren, (Fig 2.4), always known as 'Jonky' (pronounced Yonky), qualified MB.BS from University College Hospital in 1934, where he worked for Sir Thomas Lewis and Sir George Pickering. While doing his house jobs he passed the MRCP in 1935 and the FRCS the following year. He regards the latter achievement as unfortunate. As assistant physician he studied the physiology of referred pain and was awarded a Beit Memorial Fellowship.

In 1939 war was imminent and hospital patients and services were transferred from London to designated sectors of the country around London in order to free up beds in the city for expected air raid casualties. Kellgren had not planned a surgical career but his Dean, noting his surgical qualification, appointed him as officer in charge of the Great Ormond Street Children's Surgical unit at Hemel Hempstead. He described the work as not very interesting being mainly the removal of tuberculous lymph nodes, hernias, correction of undescended testicles and the like. He transferred to the Professorial Surgical Unit at a tuberculosis hospital, Leavesden, in Abbots Langley as first assistant to Professor Pilcher who was developing chest surgery. Kellgren undertook surgery for prolapsed intervertebral discs. Surgery for the survivors of the Dunkirk evacuation interrupted this work and in 1941 he joined the Royal Army Medical Corps and was posted to front line work in North Africa where he took part in the landing at Algiers and the Tunisian campaign.

It was perhaps lucky for him that the authorities were unaware that through a family connection he spoke demotic Russian- otherwise he might have found himself posted to liaise with the Red Army!

After the landings his field hospital was delegated to look after soldiers of the Free French army, assisted by two French surgical teams. The hospital was sited in an ancient Carthaginian city. Disaster to the hospital team struck when it was ordered to pack up and be ready to move. But no movement order arrived. So things continued in enforced idleness in the sand and heat of the desert for many months. Team morale was broken and never really returned. Eventually an officer went back to HQ on the weekly lorry that brought water and mail, only to find that the team was thought to be already in Sicily!

After a year doing little he was posted to a casualty clearing station with the Indian forces in Italy, thence Naples. With demobilisation he returned to the UK after five years of surgery with the problem of how to plan his future career. He did not want to be a London surgeon (income all at that time derived from private practice). He consulted the Secretary of the Medical Research Council (Mellanby) and was recommended to work with Herbert Seddon at the Wingfield Morris (now Nuffield) Orthopaedic Hospital in Oxford. At that time he was studying peripheral nerve injuries and the effects of cooling on pain perception.

Manchester was lucky in that it had in 1946 as Vice Chancellor Sir John (later Lord) Stopford. He had been professor of anatomy, a brilliant teacher who had done excellent research on the sympathetic nervous system. As Chairman of The Nuffield Foundation he arranged for The Foundation to grant the University of Manchester £10,000 annually for ten years to establish 'The University of Manchester Centre for Research into Chronic Rheumatism'. It was to have clinical and pathology sections. Eric Bywaters had been approached for the clinical section but did not wish to leave London. In the summer of 1947 Kellgren received a letter from Prof Robert Platt inviting him to apply for the job. He did, and was appointed.

The Centre for Research into Chronic Rheumatism was seen from the start as 'multi-disciplinary'. Prof. SL Baker, who had described a rare disease of bone collagen, and Dr John Ball were the first two pathologists. Research started on the then widely held premise that rheumatology was concerned with diseases of the connective tissue system. David Jackson and John Scott (later at Taplow) tackled the problems of connective tissue biochemistry. Buick Slack, an early collector of Lowry paintings, was the research fellow who did some of the first radiocarbon collagen turnover studies. A rheumatology study group that included colleagues from other faculties met weekly.

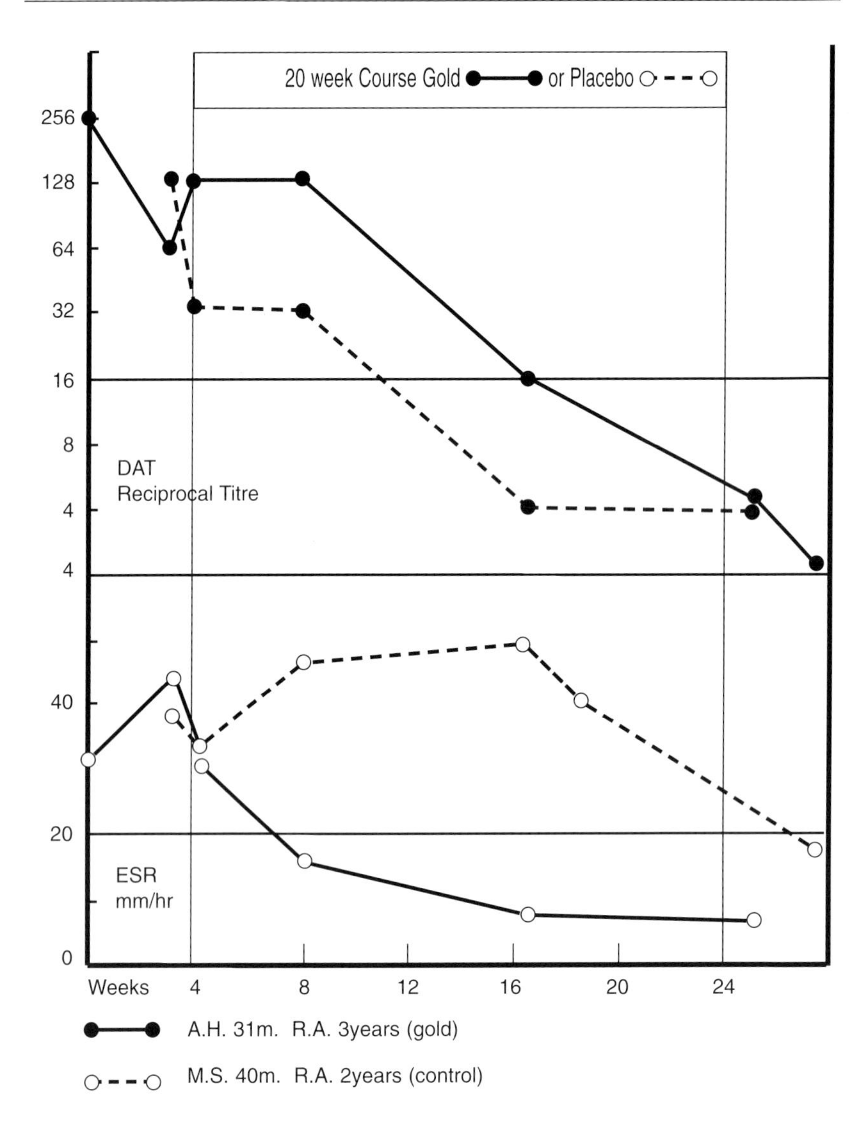

Fig 2.5. rheumatoid arthritis. Similar responces to gold treatment and placebo. ESR = Erythrocyte sedimentation rate. DAT = Differential agglutination titre for rheumatoid factor

Biophysics was not available in Manchester at the time so collaboration was arranged with Prof Astbury, a fibre chemist in Leeds, for electron microscopy studies. The first of these was on fibrinoid and showed, inter alia, that the change of collagen to fibrinoid was unaffected by corticosteroid treatment and that fibrinoid was just collagen coated with fibrin.

In 1952 Lord Stopford arranged a visit by members of the Nuffield committee. They were sufficiently impressed to continue and increase their grant, and in 1953 Stopford persuaded the Arthritis and Rheumatism Council to endow the first UK Chair of Rheumatology at a salary of £4,000 *per annum*. Kellgren was appointed Professor and head of an established University Department with lecturers in clinical medicine, pathology, biochemistry and biophysics. All staff had teaching commitments in their respective disciplines.

Clinicians of the Unit took part in the multicentre comparison of cortisone and aspirin in rheumatoid arthritis with Professor Bradford Hill as statistician. Later there was a trial comparing gold treatment with placebo injections. This confirmed that gold was more effective than placebo in inducing remissions of rheumatoid arthritis but also showed some remarkable remissions in the placebo arm of the trial. (Figure 2.5)

Dr John Popert was in charge of a trial of the anti-malarial drug chloroquine phosphate that showed that it could induce remissions in rheumatoid arthritis and could reduce the titre of circulating rheumatoid factor more than did gold therapy. When appointed as rheumatologist at Droitwich Popert continued to champion the use of anti-malarials in rheumatoid arthritis.

A Miners' Welfare Commission had existed in Lancashire from about 1936 and in January 1948 the Rheumatic Disease Research Centre was approached by the Commission asking that Kellgren should look into the problems of rheumatism in miners. The Professor of Occupational Medicine, Ronnie Lane, whose office was in the next corridor, gave advice. The Miners' Welfare Commission funded the appointment of John Lawrence who based his work on the Miners' clinic at Walkden. The answer to the problem lay in the terrible conditions under which the miners had to work in the Lancashire pits. The coal seams were between 4 and 5 feet high, neither high enough to stand up nor so low that they had to crawl. The seams that determined the floors on which the miners stood sloped at up to 45°. The results were damage to backs, hips, and knees from the working position forced on them.

The study of the miners led to a population study of the prevalence of rheumatic diseases. Janet Aitken-Swan was seconded from Prof. Lane's department to

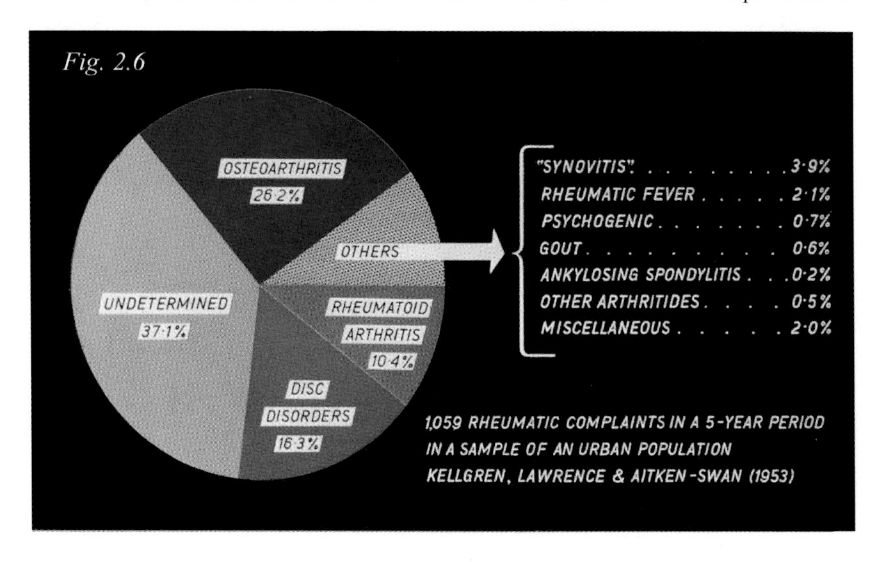

Fig. 2.6

assist John Lawrence. The first population survey of rheumatic complaints was based on the town of Leigh in Lancashire and used house-sampling survey techniques supported by clinical, radiological and serological assessments. It was published in 1953 (Kellgren, Lawrence and Aitken-Swan, 1953) (Figure 2.6). Lawrence continued to work in the Walkden clinic for some years, comparing the rheumatic complaints of the mining face workers with those of the engineers and clerical workers. The pain threshold of the miners was exceptionally high. Despite formidable spinal changes on x-ray, the miner with an obvious limp, back stiffness and missing ankle reflexes might only say he was 'a bit hangy like'. In contrast the engineers and clerical workers with lesser x-ray lesions were more vocal. The psychology of pain perception and the influence of motivation on complaint threshold still have much to tell.

There was also a fruitful collaboration between the Rheumatic Diseases Research Centre in Manchester and the Pneumoconiosis Research Unit in Llandough under the direction of Archie Cochrane. Caplan's Syndrome, a characteristic appearance on chest X-ray of pneumoconiosis (Figure 2.7) in miners who had, *or who were destined to develop,* rheumatoid arthritis formed an important link. This led to a comprehensive clinical, X-ray and serological survey of miners and of a control population of men aged 49-59 in the Vale of Glamorgan.

The science base of rheumatology at Manchester was thus divided between epidemiology and connective tissue biochemistry, along with descriptive studies of morbid anatomy based on the work of Dr John Ball. The temptation to follow other centres into immunology was avoided. Data were collected on the complications of rheumatoid arthritis such as the association with 'honeycomb lung'. Dr James Sharp's collaboration with the Manchester Eye Hospital next door to the Royal Infirmary alerted

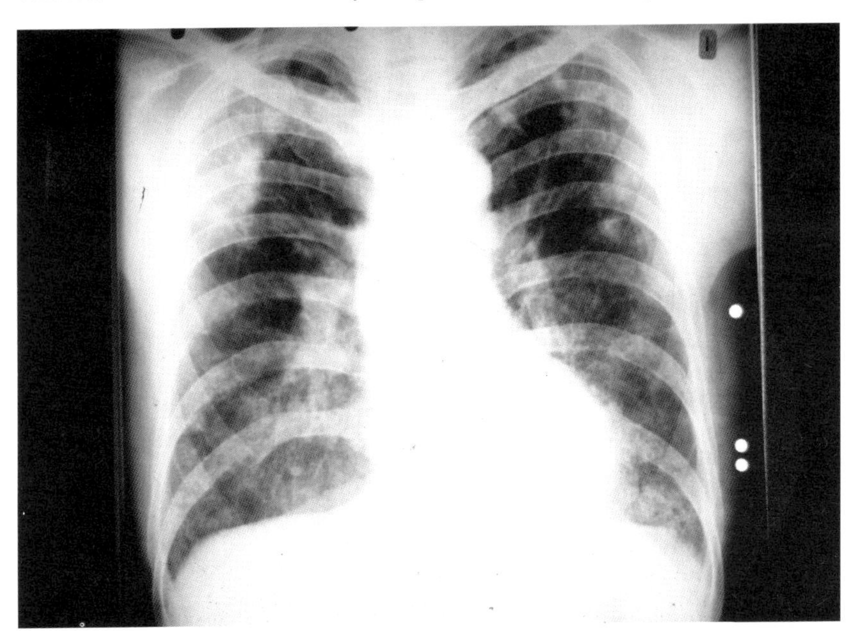

Fig 2.7. Chest Xray of Caplan's Syndrome

ophthalmologists everywhere to the need to screen all iritis and uveitis patients for signs of ankylosing spondylitis and related diseases.

From the early days of his appointment Kellgren had kept departmental records of all patients seen and diagnoses made. These were separate from the records held by the hospital, which tended like most hospital records to the chaotic. A review of those who were labelled 'Polyarthritis, Atypical', usually because of unusual distribution of joint involvement and persistently negative tests for rheumatoid factor, revealed some rarities like reticulohistiocytosis, but more importantly it documented the appearance of psoriatic polyarthritis sometimes years before the appearance of the psoriasis. Conversely some of those with persistently seronegative polyarthritis might convert to seropositive if followed for long enough.

There were ten rheumatology beds in the Manchester Royal Infirmary, at first in a surgical and later in a medical ward, where patients could be investigated. Patients were later transferred to the Devonshire Royal Hospital (DRH) at Buxton where Dr Ronnie Harris was the Director of Rehabilitation and Dr Stuart Barber was Physician with an interest in rheumatology.

In the early days, coming from a largely surgical background, Kellgren was greatly helped by Dr Oscar Janus, appointed as Lecturer in Clinical Rheumatology but in fact an excellent general physician who was destined to become Consultant in General Medicine at Oldham. Dr James Sharp joined as Senior Lecturer in 1951 and was joined by the author in 1956.

Clinics serviced from the Rheumatism Research Centre had been held at the nearby Christie Hospital at the request of its Director, Dr Ralston-Patterson, since 1948. Their job was to advise on the management of ankylosing spondylitis (AS) patients referred for radiotherapy. In the UK at that time, AS patients were often treated by orthopaedic surgeons along the same lines as they would treat tuberculous disease of the spine, namely by rest and immobilisation. Some sufferers were confined to plaster beds and 'Swain's Corsets', emerging later as statues. In the 1950's radiotherapy had been shown to help AS back pain and became the standard treatment for this disease until it was realised that the patients could get equal if not better relief from phenylbutazone without the risks of radiotherapy. Kellgren taught that AS sufferers did badly with rest and improved with movement, a teaching that was later to inspire the formation of the National Ankylosing Spondylitis Society (NASS).

The association with the AS clinic led to early attempts at corrective osteotomy for fixed flexion deformity of the neck. On one occasion a patient who had been anaesthetised and whose airway had been intubated was being turned over so that the surgeon Mr Lloyd-Griffiths could operate on the back of the neck. There was an ominous crack as the stiffened neck broke. The operation was abandoned. The neck and head were fixed in a Minerva Splint in the new position. The patient not only survived but did very well and was grateful, but doubtless impressed at how the work was done without leaving a scar!

There was also a big programme of work on atlanto-axial subluxation in rheumatoid arthritis and its neurological complications, that was presented to the Association of Physicians.

It had been Kellgren's policy to limit the number of clinical trainees on fellowships and junior jobs because of the then shortage of openings for rheumatology consultants. Those who passed through the Centre for Chronic Rheumatic Diseases in trainee positions and who stayed in rheumatology in the UK incuded John Popert (Droitwich), Dennis Pitkeithly (Glasgow), Maurice Jeffery (Harrogate), Peter Smith (North Manchester) and Tom Chalmers (Edinburgh)

Meanwhile Kellgren was becoming increasingly involved in University administration. In 1961 he had been appointed Dean of Postgraduate studies for a five-year period. During this time postgraduate centres were established and postgraduate tutors appointed in all of the 22 district general hospitals in the region. When this task was over he was appointed University member of the Manchester Regional Hospital Board and Chairman of the Board's medical advisory committee. The enlargement of the medical school from 100 to 275 students involved the development of two additional teaching hospitals in South Manchester and Salford, incurring endless planning committees and the appointment of a raft of additional professors. At first Kellgren could manage his clinical as well as his administrative responsibilities but in 1968 a crisis occurred. Kellgren had accepted to be Dean of the Medical School and later pro-Vice Chancellor. As such he had to cope with student riots in which the medics and engineers had to steady the boat.

Kellgren had relied on his colleague Tom Chalmers, to 'manage the shop' from the clinical point of view. But Chalmers wanted to move back to Edinburgh and did so after one year. His post was advertised and Dr Lennox Holt from Hammersmith Hospital was appointed. They were large shoes to step into. Some of his older colleagues were disappointed with the change in the scientific approach and most of the original research team dispersed.

In 1973 Kellgren undertook further administrative responsibilities with the formalities of the opening of the Stopford Building. When Kellgren retired in 1977 it was decided to move the direction of Manchester academic rheumatology to the Hope Hospital in Salford and Dr Malcolm Jayson, previously at Bath and Bristol, was elected Professor.

The remaining clinical service at the Manchester Royal Infirmary was increased by the appointment of Dr Robert Bernstein from Hammersmith Hospital as Holt's colleague. The net effect was considerably to enlarge the rheumatology presence in Greater Manchester, based now on the Hope Hospital, with satellite centres at the Manchester Royal Infirmary, the Osteoarticular pathology service and the Arthritis and Rheumatism Council's Epidemiological Research Unit.

Exceptionally amongst UK academic rheumatologists, Jayson has taken a special interest in back pain. In Bristol he had worked with a physiotherapist, Sue Young, to compare conventional treatment of back pain with the results of manipulation by the Maitland technique. His textbook entitled 'The Lumbar Spine and Back Pain' (1976), has been updated through three further editions. He has explored the effects of venous obstruction and oedema of nerve root ganglia[3] and fibrosis in the nerve root

3 First described by Bradford and Spurling in 1941 (see Chapter 8 and Figure 8.1.)

canals in connection with chronic back pain syndromes. Jayson became President of the International Society for the Study of the Lumbar spine. He retired from administrative work in 1996 but continues part time in his department.

Dr Tony Freemont (Professor of Osteoarticular Pathology) has taken over as Head of Department. With Dr Philipe Goupille he is taking the study of back pain syndromes further, looking at vascular endothelial damage, cytokine release and nerve fibre changes. The department's beds have fallen from 65 to 28, with further reductions foreseen. Despite this the in-patient turnover rate has doubled. There are outpatient sessions for ankylosing spondylitis sufferers. Dr Terry O'Neil provides a clinical osteoporosis service and undertakes epidemiological research in cooperation with Prof. Alan Silman. A programme of clinical study and research into systemic sclerosis is under the supervision of Dr Ariane Herrick.

There is a new look at relaxin, the hormone that relaxes the pelvic ligaments in women prior to giving birth. The development of genetically engineered relaxin has enabled larger doses to be given than were available 40 years previously when this was first tried without success.

Skin wounds in a foetus heal without scarring. Starting from this observation research into antibodies to the Transforming Growth Factor family (TGF-1&2) has indicated that there may be a method for stopping the excessive fibrosis in systemic sclerosis.

Manchester paediatric rheumatology was first organised by Dr Holt at the Booth Hall Hospital. Another service was set up at Pendlebury Hospital. It was planned to combine them when a new paediatric hospital is built. Physical Medicine does not have a large presence in Manchester. Drs Peter Copp and Janet Keenan do electromyography for carpal tunnel and peripheral nerve problems. Another service also based on the Manchester Royal Infirmary was run by the neurophysiologists. Neurosurgery, neurophysiology and neurology were in process of being gathered together at the Hope Hospital. Rehabilitation had become largely a province of neurology, although the Devonshire Royal Hospital at Buxton, originally planned for closure in 1999, continued to act as a decanting hospital for the Royal Infirmary rheumatology patients.

Prof. Jayson set up the 'Manchester and Salford Back Pain Centre' and with Dr Anthony Jones this expanded to study all aspects of pain perception, including brain imaging by computerised electroencephalograhic and positron emission scanning.

About fifty trainees in rheumatology have passed through the Manchester rheumatology service during Jayson's time and of these five have become professors. All district hospitals in the North West Health Region now have a least one rheumatologist on the consultant staff.

JJR. Duthie and the Rheumatic Diseases Research Unit at Edinburgh

John James Reid Duthie, always known as Ian, was born on the 2nd of October 1911. He trained in medicine in Aberdeen, qualifying in 1933. It is likely that one of his teachers was John McMichael, at that time Senior Lecturer in Aberdeen and later Professor of Medicine at the Postgraduate Medical School, Hammersmith Hospital. After qualification Duthie was steered towards rheumatology by his professor, Sir Stanley Davidson, and in preparation for this he visited other rheumatology centres in the UK including George Kersley at Bath. A Travelling Fellowship took him to the USA and the Robert Breck Brigham hospital in Boston for further experience.

After war started in 1939, Dr Frank Howitt, who had been the first President of the Heberden Society and a senior figure in Physical Medicine, was asked to select a team of consultants who could oversee rehabilitation services for the army. Duthie was among those chosen, and a photograph published in 'Rheumatology and Rehabilitation' by Kersley and Glyn (1991) shows him [figure 2.8] as a member of the team. Duthie, with his army cap awry, and his uniform rather crumpled, clearly was not a strong believer in military 'spit and polish'. He served from 1940 to1946 after which he was appointed as Senior Lecturer in Medicine at Edinburgh, under the professorship of Sir Stanley Davidson who had moved from Aberdeen. Davidson asked Duthie to set up a Bone and Joint Research Unit in the Northern General Hospital, an institution that had been the isolation hospital for Leith, before Leith became part of Edinburgh.

At that time the Unit consisted of 'Two pavilion type wards together with one or two meagre rooms for consultations and a secretary in an outlying hut – relic of a first world war annex, distant from the wards and with no covered access from them' (Alan Hill).

But things were to get better. The 1955 Report of the Nuffield Foundation reads: "The principle event (in 1955) has been the completion and opening of the Oliver Bird Building to house the clinical and laboratory research of the Rheumatic Unit, Northern General Hospital, Edinburgh, under Dr JJR Duthie. In the presence of Captain Oliver Bird, M.C., the new building was opened on the 23rd of April 1955 by Lord Strathclyde, Minister of State for Scotland. The building, designed by Mr J Holt,

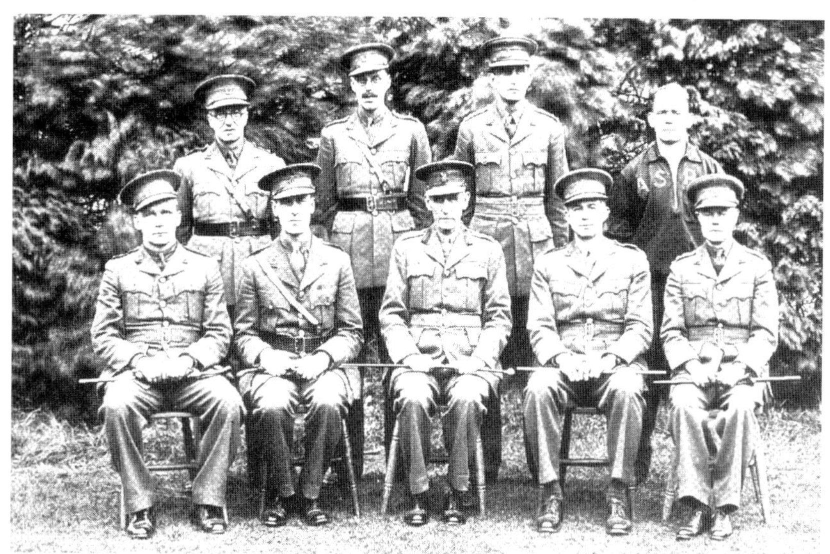

Fig 2.8. Ian Duthie in uniform (sitting left).

consists of two single story blocks connected by a glass link which forms the entrance hall. The plan is L-shaped and the main section contains six consulting rooms each equipped with an examination couch, wash-basin, built-in blood-pressure machines and X-ray viewing-boxes. A waiting space open to the corridor is in the centre of the consulting area, with dressing-cubicles and toilets adjoining. Two laboratories and a conference room are at the end of this block; the laboratories have metal unit fitments that can be interchanged or added to later. There is also a small animal-house."

An additional grant of £65,750 over 5 years was promised to help with running costs and research.

"The addition of the Oliver Bird Building transformed these basic facilities into a well laid out clinic, laboratory, library and offices- all I think now demolished and replaced by a supermarket" –(Hill, 1998)

Duthie rapidly built up his unit assisted at first by Drs RJ (Jack) Sinclair and WRM (Rowland) Alexander. Sinclair was lead author of a much cited study of the bone, joint and visceral problems of Marfan's syndrome. Alexander was a key figure in the early studies on the anaemia of rheumatoid arthritis. The Unit had the reputation and Duthie had the personality to attract many capable staff and research Fellows. Research grants from local and national funding organisations accompanied them. Gardner described Duthie as "A perceptive and sensitive but direct physician who did not waste words". Hill recalls him as "An inspiring team leader and his research conferences were particularly lively, uninhibited, and stimulating, he thrived on debate and argument". Hill, seeming unintentionally to mix his dog similies, writes: "in the pursuit of any line of investigation he would seize it in his teeth like a terrier and never let go, which chimed with his undergraduate prowess as a boxer". "He appeared to be the archetypal Aberdonian, overtly honest, frank, outspoken, intolerant of the idle or disinterested" (Gardner).

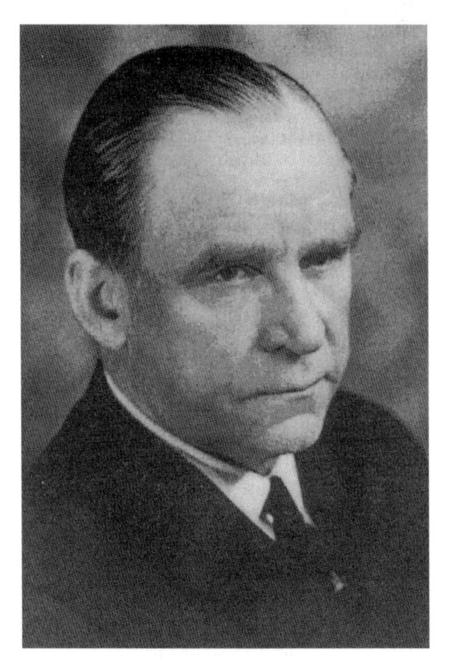

Fig 2.9. Professor JJR Duthie

Duthie (Figure 2.9) was an excellent Chairman of the Research Committee of the Arthritis and Rheumatism Council (ARC), decisive yet kindly and enlightened. Dr AJ Collins was a pharmacologist at Bath University who applied for funds to investigate inflammatory kinins at a time when the Committee interviewed applicants. Duthie and the Committee liked the proposer but not the proposal and said they would support him if he took six months off to learn more about kinins under the expert tuition of Professor Keele of the Middlesex Hospital. This done, Collins returned to Bath, took a medical degree and subsequently made important observations on the action of non-steroidal anti-inflammatory drugs on the gastro-intestinal tract in man. It is doubtful if this would have happened under another chairman, or current ARC practice, which is to judge the application but not interview the applicant.

Duthie's research interests were many. On his return from the USA he wrote an account of his experiences in the first volume of the Annals of Rheumatic Diseases. He was impressed with the social and home service departments set up to help the transition of the patient from hospital to home, the highly trained young women who ran them, the Occupational Therapy services and the organisation of an arthritis unit. (Duthie, 1939). His association with John Richmond, Jack Sinclair, Rowland Alexander, Dugald Gardner and others led to a series of papers, eleven in all, on aspects of the anaemia of rheumatoid arthritis. The first of these was published in 1949 (Sinclair and Duthie, 1949). Of two other papers published in 1956 with colleagues one concerned the survival of transfused erythrocytes in patients with rheumatoid arthritis. The other described sternal marrow studies in 60 patients in 41 % of whom no iron was detected by the Prussian blue method, but all had iron detected chemically.

Some of the earlier investigations of the anaemia of rheumatoid arthritis may have been flawed. Treatment of the disease at that time was firmly under American influence that proclaimed that large doses of aspirin were 'mandatory' in rheumatoid arthritis. The Unit was aware that aspirin could cause gastrointestinal bleeding but relied on non-quantitative fecal occult blood tests to detect it. The accurate radio-chromium-labelled red cell method was not introduced until about 1957. The earlier studies could not take account of the extent to which symtomless aspirin-induced gastro-intestinal bleeding might have modified the findings.

Duthie's concern with sociological issues led to the setting up, (with help from The Nuffield Foundation), of an industrial rheumatology unit with Dr Jock Anderson looking at the different patterns of back pain and other rheumatic complaints and correlating these with occupation. His unit also studied the experimental production of nodules, the nature of rheumatoid arthritis cells, the search for infective agents, the study of iron metabolism in this disease and therapeutic trials of likely candidate drugs. When he was nearing retirement, he gave the impression that his passion was to find a cure for rheumatoid arthritis and he started using combinations of drugs. It was as though he had to move quickly in the time that was left him.

Duthie sensed that an obscure infection might be the cause of rheumatoid arthritis. It had to be discovered or ruled out. He worked with Dr S. Stewart on mycoplasmata but was cautious about the diphtheroid bacilli that Dr Stewart grew from some synovial tissues. Their significance as cause or harmless 'bystander' remains controversial. However it did lead him to co-operate with Professor Marrion of the University Department of Microbiology in a series of experiments attempting to transmit rheumatoid arthritis to baboons, with negative results.

An interesting observation that was published with co-author LH Truelove (Truelove and Duthie, 1959)) concerned a specific effect of aspirin in suppressing the vasodilating skin reaction to the tetrahydro furfuryl ester of nicotinic acid. Later he was to suggest that, confronted with a comatose patient, the suppression of this skin reaction could be used to confirm aspirin poisoning. An important and early part of the Unit's work was collaboration with orthopaedic surgeons, particularly Douglas Saville and Willy Souttar at the Princess Margaret Rose hospital.

Duthie was not afraid to experiment on himself. He antedated Hollander in putting a thermocouple into a knee (his own) to measure changes in intra-articular temperature. More dangerous, although the danger could not have been anticipated at the time, was an experiment with synovial fluid. He had shown that the intradermal injection of synovial fluid from a rheumatoid arthritis patient led to a delayed skin reaction both in healthy individuals and in other patients with rheumatoid arthritis. However, cell-free fluids did not provoke a reaction. During these experiments he used as a control for synovial fluid, ascitic fluid from a patient with cirrhosis of the liver. This led to an outbreak of hepatitis from which he too suffered. There were three fatalities. The only good thing to come out of this was that it did yield precise data on the incubation period of this particular kind of hepatitis. These findings were not published in the medical press but the data were sent privately to people with a special interest in liver disease.(Alan Hill)

Unlike his contemporaries, Bywaters and Kellgren, he believed that prolonged rest was essential for inflamed joints. Accordingly his patients were put though particularly demanding regimes of bed-rest and splinting. He did not seek to limit the numbers of UK rheumatologists he trained because of the shortage of consultant posts. In the 1940s and 1950s there were few openings for young rheumatologists. But Scotland has always had a tradition of exporting doctors. In the event he was justified. As the members of his team progressed to consultant status, vacancies became available as the older physical medicine specialists retired. The more enlightened teaching hospitals, faced with decreasing admissions for infection-related diseases, realised that rheumatology was a field of medicine that was shrugging off its traditional physical medicine and spa image. Early Hammersmith UK trainees went almost exclusively to hospitals in London but the 'Duthie Diaspora' scattered his UK trainees to posts all over the country and abroad.

Those who trained with Duthie (and where they went in the UK) included Jack Sinclair, Rowland Alexander, Tom Chalmers, and John McCormick (who stayed in or returned to Edinburgh), Alan Hill, (Stoke Mandeville), Dugald Gardner, (Director of the Kennedy Institute), Malcolm Thompson, (Newcastle), Alistair Mowat, (Oxford), Jock Anderson, (Community Medicine at Guy's Hospital), Gabriel Panayi, (Guy's), Ted Hothersall, (North Staffs), Ted Sever, (Northampton), Alex Lawson, (Dunfermline), Trevor Constable, (Walsal), Clifford Eastmond, (Aberdeen), Nigel Dunn, (Hartlepool), and Joan Bremner, (Manchester epidemiology).

Following the retirement of Duthie in 1977 there was an interregnum while Tom Chalmers was in charge. He was succeeded by Prof. George Nuki, (Figure 2.10) previously at Cardiff and Glasgow, and for whom Duthie's university-funded Professorial Chair was taken over and endowed by the Arthritis and Rheumatism Council.

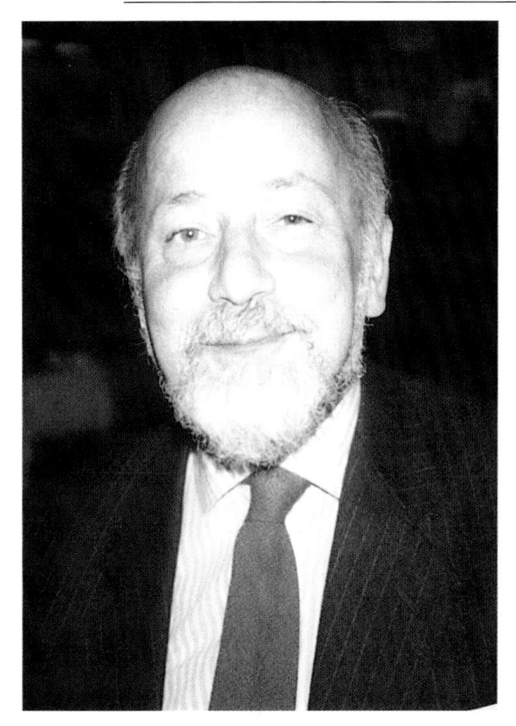

Fig 2.10. Prof George Nuki.

There followed a rearrangement and rationalisation of the rheumatism unit. The buildings at the Northern General Hospital, by then over twenty years old, were abandoned and the rheumatology unit transferred to the Western General Infirmary where all academic activity took place. Within the academic unit the staff were sub-specialised. Thus Nuki 'looked after' cartilage cell biology, osteoarthritis and gout, Nigel Hurst dealt with outcome measures and priority setting, Mike Lambert with health economics, Raashid Luqmani with vasculitis and Veena Dhillon with osteoporosis and health services research. All the academic rheumatologists had rheumatology commitments at the peripheral hospitals as well. The services for the city and the surrounding district general hospitals were organised on the 'Hub and Spokes' plan. None of the peripheral hospitals had independent staff, but those who worked there did naturally develop their local loyalties. The situation differed from the Yorkshire region where all the District General Hospitals had independent rheumatologists, although associated with the University-linked Leeds General Hospital through regional Rheumatology Clinical Societies.

The Scottish Rheumatology Club covered the whole of Scotland including the Highlands and Islands, (which looked to Inverness and Aberdeen for their services). Meetings were held twice a year, one in the Western General Infirmary and one in the hospital of the most recently appointed rheumatologist.

Nuki considered that his patients 'got the best surgical rheumatology service in the country' with the support of Prof. Abernethy (orthopaedics), Geoff Hooper (hand surgery), Mike McMaster, (spinal surgery). There was a long tradition of co-operation with the Princess Margaret Rose Orthopaedic hospital, going back to Willy Soutar and others. Soutar had now retired but the Soutar Elbow was still the leading elbow prosthesis. Richie Nutton had investigated shoulder prostheses and was exploring the possibilities of imaging soft tissue lesions using nuclear magnetic resonance. The surgeons used a variety of prostheses for knee replacements.

The surgical work was backed up by experimental animal research. Melvin Pond, a veterinarian studying rupture of the anterior cruciate ligament in dogs, had shown that this was followed by osteoarthritis unless the ligament was mended. Experimental section of the ligament (which could be done with a fine ophthalmic scalpel without opening the joint) was also followed by osteoarthritis and had become the standard animal model for this disease. The model had been used for testing experimental synovial fluids. However, even when these possessed the same viscoelastic properties as natural fluid, they were scavenged from the joint by the synovial membrane in a few days, confirming previous work by Dr Ian Haslock at South Cleveland. The model was also used by Helen Muir, head of biochemistry at the Kennedy Institute, studying the composition of cartilage in health and disease.

In the 1950s Paul Weiss, a Chicago embryologist, was working on the way in which the mechanical condition of a culture medium, whether stretched or compressed, could profoundly influence the direction of cell growth within it. In an interesting co-operation with Dr DMO Wright (Department of Physiology) and colleagues, rheumatology research at Edinburgh was studying the response of chondrocytes to mechanical strains of the culture medium. The work was relevant to cartilage atrophy in paralysed limbs. Abnormal responses had already been found in osteoarthritic cartilage.

A paediatric rheumatology service in Edinburgh begun by Tom Chalmers had been expanded by Raashid Luqmani. In Scotland paediatric rheumatology was mostly looked after by a combination of an 'adult' rheumatologist and a paediatrician with inpatients in a children's hospital. Nuki considered that in future there would be one specialist paediatric rheumatologist for the region, to create a nucleus of expertise and train up a cadre of specialist paediatricians to take on paediatric rheumatology in the periphery.

Soon after his appointment, Nuki took advantage of the presence in Edinburgh of facilities for whole body scanning using radio-calcium to measure bone density. This method used fairly high fluxes of ionising radiation and the scanner required was not commonly available. As it was both quantitative and specific for calcium it could be seen as the gold standard against which methods such as dual x-ray absorptiometry (DXA) could be judged. Nuki and his colleagues were able to distinguish the loss of body calcium caused by rheumatoid arthritis and polymyalgia rheumatica from the additional loss caused by corticosteroid therapy.

Prof. Bill Gillespie, an orthopaedic surgeon who believed in the clinical trial method applied to surgical procedures, had started a large randomised prospective multi-centre MRC-funded controlled trial of Vitamin D using as outcome measure fracture of the femoral neck.

A special interest of the Edinburgh service had been Community Rheumatology. The late Dr Andy Martynoga had been Senior Registrar at the Northern General Hospital. Following his training in rheumatology he went into general practice. But he had a vision of the work of 'Community Rheumatologist' and in the event was appointed as such in Fife. The appointment was successful and reduced the need for long distance referrals of patients with difficult and complicated disease. After Martynoga's death Jane Gibson, (trained at Northwick Park and Manchester) took on the job. She visits the Western General Infirmary once or twice a year.

At one time the Arthritis and Rheumatism Council was concerned that expertise in osteoarticular morbid anatomy, in the tradition of Dr Douglas Collins at

Harrogate, might disappear in this country. Dr John Ball at Manchester had died and Dr. Dugald Gardner had retired from the Kennedy Institute. Nuki persuaded the Council to appoint Gardner as Proleptic Professor of Osteoarticular Pathology in Edinburgh. He in turn trained Donald Salter.

Chapter 3. Developments in the London Teaching Hospitals

The benefactions of the Arthritis and Rheumatism Council and of the Oliver Bird Fund of the Nuffield Foundation together with the example of the three academic units at Hammersmith, Manchester and Edinburgh ensured that the knowledge of what rheumatology had to offer began to spread across the country. At the same time there was a gradual conversion of consultant posts in physical medicine to consultant posts in rheumatology. The changes took place in different places at different rates. There were those who opposed it. Some of these were physical medicine specialists who were proud of their traditions. After all, it was Sir Robert Stanton Woods who was the first to have the title Consultant in Physical Medicine and who had been knighted for the services he gave to royalty. Physical medicine specialists had spearheaded rehabilitation services for the armed services in both world wars. They had set up a separate British Association for Physical Medicine in 1943, partly to balance the more narrowly targeted Heberden Society. In 1944 they had negotiated for the Diploma in Physical Medicine. It was a diploma that some younger rheumatologists such as Eric Hamilton at Kings College Hospital felt constrained to take to establish credentials to get a consultant job. Moreover they were in a strong position. They were the sitting tenants. They were the alternatives for patients with rheumatic diseases who did not get sent to the spa hospitals. The committees that in those days ran the hospitals consisted only of medically qualified staff. The physical medicine specialist was the doctor who could speak for the occupational therapy and physiotherapy departments on those committees.

Some physical medicine specialists were not particularly concerned. One cause of lack of coherence among them was that they tended to be jacks of all trades within the hospital because their work had diversified in many ways. At St Thomas's, Phillipe Bauwens had pioneered electromyography and James Cyriax had developed a system of spinal manipulation which still has many followers. Others such as Philip Nichols at the Mary Marlborough Lodge at the Nuffield Hospital in Oxford had a vision of how peacetime rehabilitation would develop. In that role physical medicine departments would deal with a wide variety of non-rheumatic physically disabled patients. There was no particular imperative for rheumatologists to take on the role of doctors in charge of physiotherapy and occupational therapy departments. A spot check at Hammersmith Hospital in 1959 showed that the major users of physiotherapy services were orthopaedic surgeons. They were followed by neurologists and respiratory disease physicians. Rheumatologists were quite a way down the list.

Opposition was also encountered from General Physicians. At that time all bed-holding physicians did general medicine as well as the specialty in which they were particularly interested. Physical medicine specialists were seldom bed-holders and within the hospital hierarchy were often regarded as second class citizens. Some of the older ones had no postgraduate qualifications. Sir Robert Stanton Woods was a rare exception. In 1936 he had been allotted six beds by the Medical Council (committee of consultants) at the London Hospital 'for the investigation and treatment of patients with rheumatic diseases'.

Logie Bain in Aberdeen exemplified the attitude prevalent at the time. He was well regarded but when appointed as consultant in Physical Medicine at Aberdeen in 1947 no beds were attached to his position, only an outpatient clinic held in the local swimming baths. In Plymouth physical medicine took place in a separate out patient building distant from the main hospitals.

Two Professors of Medicine were indifferent to the development of rheumatology and did not in their hospitals actively encourage it. Their hospitals were seen as 'black holes' for rheumatology in the early days. Paradoxically both had been connected to the Heberden Society. Professor Bruce Perry (Bristol) had been interested in rheumatic fever and rheumatic heart disease. He was a founder member of the Empire Rheumatism Council and had joined the Heberden Society for a while. Later he set up an ankylosing spondylitis clinic that he devolved to Dr Harry West. He may have considered that he sufficiently represented rheumatology in Bristol and in any case could not or did not wish to set up a system in competition with Bath.

Sir Henry, later Lord, Cohen had been President of the Heberden Society from 1950 to 1952, after that its Roundsman and Orator. Again, as a general physician with an interest in rheumatic diseases he may have felt that there was no need for a specialist rheumatology service in Liverpool. He may also have been influenced by the Liverpool orthopaedic surgeons. They were particularly strong in that city, under Sir Robert Jones, Thomas McMurray, JS Armour and Reginald Watson-Jones and they saw the bulk of chronic rheumatic problems referred to hospital.

Even where rheumatology was accepted as an important service for patients the main hospitals tended to keep it at a distance. This had advantages if the place chosen was a 'green field site', free from the restrictions of the traditional hospital hierarchy and with space and funds to develop. Thus in Edinburgh, rheumatology had been devolved to a converted isolation hospital. In Glasgow the academic rheumatology service under Dr Watson Buchanan was sited in a condemned tuberculosis hospital in Baird Street opposite slum tenements. In Leeds the rheumatology service was housed in a small Victorian villa in Clarendon Road near to the University, but some distance from the Infirmary. Perhaps the best solution was to have rheumatology alongside the services of a recently established small general hospital, as at the Canadian Red Cross Memorial Hospital at Taplow or the converted wartime Emergency Medical Services (EMS) hospital at Stoke Mandeville, to share diagnostic facilities and ensure that other expertise was easily available.

The London Teaching Hospitals

There were thirteen London teaching hospitals at the end of the war. A series of mergers, usually staunchly resisted, were to reduce this by 1998 to five teaching hospital trusts and five combined medical schools with unwieldy names. The West London Hospital, a minnow compared with the others, was subsumed by Charing Cross Hospital in 1965 and later closed. University College, Middlesex and Royal Free Hospital medical schools formed one merger. Kings went in with Guy's and St Thomas's medical schools. St Bartholomew's and The (by then *Royal)* London Hospital became The Royal Hospitals Trust. A brand new preclinical medical school was developed at Imperial College, part of the Imperial College of Science, Technology and Medicine that included St Mary's, Charing Cross, the rebuilt Chelsea and Westminster undergraduate medical schools and the post graduate medical schools at Hammersmith and Northwick Park. Only St George's, by then in Tooting, escaped.

The United Medical Schools of Guy's, St Thomas's and King's College Hospitals

Rheumatology at *St Thomas' Hospital* evolved out of the Department of Physical Medicine that in 1948 featured Dr Phillipe Bauwens who pioneered electrodiagnosis and electrotherapy, and Dr James Cyriax, a charismatic man who offered his services as Orthopaedic Physician. Cyriax introduced caudal epidurals and made sound anatomy-based observations on shoulder lesions. He held systematised ideas about the diagnosis and treatment of back pain about which he did not like to be questioned. In 1959 he employed a secretary to help compile a research report, based on an analysis of his patients who had had spinal manipulations, that he hoped would prove the principles of his method. It seems it never saw the light of day, nevertheless there are still practitioners who are influenced by his teachings. Dr Desmond Newton working as Chief Assistant initiated the interest of the St Thomas's Physical Medicine department in the rheumatic diseases. Newton was later appointed Consultant in Middlesbrough.

Dr DAH ('Tony') Yates succeeded Bauwens in 1966, after training at St Thomas's and Hammersmith, and Cyriax was succeeded by Dr John Mathews. Together they continued the St Thomas' interest in back pain as well as doing general rheumatology. Yates studied factors affecting the prognosis of nerve root lesions in sciatica and the medical aspects of spinal stenosis. Mathews and Yates developed epidural myelography and Mathews (1969) used the technique to demonstrate reduction of a lumbar disc prolapse following spinal manipulation and conducted controlled trials of manipulation and traction in back pain. They developed a department where all aspects of rheumatology, including paediatric and surgical rheumatology, were available for training students.

The partnership of Yates and Matthews continued until it was decided to appoint a third consultant. Only five sessions could be offered but this was not a problem for Dr Graham Hughes. He was Consultant Senior Lecturer at Hammersmith Hospital and he had been awarded £1/2m and 5 years further support from the Rothschild Foundation, together with a personal Chair, to continue his work on Systemic Lupus Erythematosis.

At Hammersmith Hughes and his colleagues had done research on the role of the anti-cardiolipin factor, based on the tendency of women with lupus to miscarry and the frequency with which lupus patients had false-positive Wasserman tests for syphilis[4]. This led to the description of the lupus anticoagulant (or anti-cardiolipin) and its contribution to a number of conditions related to venous and arterial thromboses, such as strokes, thrombocytopaenia and recurrent abortion. The varied manifestations were brought together as a syndrome (Hughes, 1998) that could underlie

4 Test reagents for syphilis that were developed in beef heart extract could detect cardiolipins. Woud be immigrants to the USA had at that time to produce a certificate showing they were free from syphilis. False positives were not infrequent and entailed refusal of a visa.

up to 16% of thrombotic strokes and 20% of instances of habitual abortion. The latter was treatable with a combination of aspirin and heparin with an 80% success rate. Hughes considered that anticardiolipin antibody might increase the risk of thrombosis in women taking oral contraceptives or hormone replacement therapy and that there was a case for screening women before they started on these hormones.

Hughes was sometimes impatient with the formalities of writing applications for research grants and in the 1980s there were occasions when he was turned down for funding. He noted that at one time he was advised by an ARC Research Committee to change his area of interest. In 1993 Hughes won the International League Against Rheumatism prize for his research. Hughes commented wryly that 'there may be some sort of lesson in the fact that this research, repeatedly turned down for funding[5], has resulted in one of the major discoveries' [of modern rheumatology]. Hughes initiated a series of workshops entitled 'Ten Topics in Rheumatology and Autoimmune Diseases' held in London and repeated in Barcelona.

Hughes' plans to take a full part in the routine work of the department were impeded as his commitments to lupus and the Lupus UK Society burgeoned. Financial stringency then decreased the number of beds available to arthritis sufferers from 20 to 6. Care for rheumatoid arthritis had increasingly to resort to out-patient treatments. The merger of Guy's and St Thomas' medical schools with departments on two sites and the Calman registrar training programme had some advantages but Yates considered that it further eroded the close integration of the department.

Yates retired in 1995 and was succeeded by Dr Tim Spector with special interests in epidemiology, osteoporosis and twins. Spector and Dr David Doyle of Whipps Cross Hospital set up the Chingford project in 1989. This was study of 1000 middle aged women screened for musculoskeletal disease and funded by the Arthritis Research Campaign. After 10 years it has yielded a number of important observations on the natural history of osteoarthritis and osteoporosis. Looking back, Yates was concerned lest the appointment of another specialist rheumatologist, while enhancing the academic output of the Department might diminish its capacity to provide training and care in the wider field of rheumatology. In this the initiatives may have moved downstream to Guy's hospital.

Guy's Hospital

During the Second World War Guy's had no named rheumatology service as such. It did have an old style Department of Physical Medicine under the direction of Dr E J ('Charlie') Crisp. A lecture from Dr Crisp on electrotherapy and massage included a discussion on the relative merits of faradic and galvanic stimulation of muscles and the abbreviations KOC and AOC, KCC and ACC, for kathode and anode opening and closing currents. The types of massage available, students were told, were effleurage, petrissage, hacking, kneading and vibration. There was no mention of rheumatic diseases. The department was 'closed', it only saw patients referred by other doctors in Guy's.

Crisp had been succeeded in 1963 by Dr Pat Kendall, an Olympic athlete

5 By no means were all of Hughes' applications unsuccessful.

who was the first to pay special attention to rheumatology. He died in 1968 and Dr Hugh Burry who had come to Guy's from New Zealand for training stayed on as Consultant in Rheumatology. Burry returned to New Zealand in 1976. Dr. Rodney Grahame qualified in 1955 from the London Hospital and entered general practice. This gave him insight into social medicine at general practitioner level. Later he trained in rheumatology at Hammersmith Hospital and the Kennedy Institute. He was appointed as Consultant Rheumatologist to Guy's Hospital in 1965 and was joined by Dr Terry Gibson in 1976. Both participated in the general medical 'Takes'. Graham dropped this in 1990 but Dr Gibson continued and is now Deputy Director of General Medicine and care of the Elderly. Dr Gibson also does a weekly clinic with nuclear medicine specialist Dr Ignac Fogelman looking after patients with osteoporosis. In 1973 the Arthritis and Rheumatism Council financed the appointment of Dr Gabriel Panayi (from Duthie's unit in Edinburgh) as ARC Lecturer. He was upgraded to Senior Lecturer in 1976. In 1990, with an endowment of £500,000 from the ARC, he was promoted to Professor.

Panayi has worked on immunogenetics and was part of the team of Woolley, Panayi and Bachelor that, simultaneously with Peter Statsny in Dallas, discovered the association of the human lymphocyte antigen HLA-DR4 with rheumatoid arthritis.

Guy's and St Thomas's medical schools merged in 1981. At first this made little difference to the clinical and academic work. In 1992 Guy's and St Thomas' Hospitals came under one Trust. Later the three medical schools of Guy's, St Thomas's and King's College Hospitals were merged (the Academic Department additionally embraced Lewisham Hospital). In 1998 the combined Academic Department received about £4.5 million annually from the Arthritis Research Campaign for all aspects of rheumatology including rheumatology in the primary care setting.

Out-patient rheumatology services continue on all three sites. The future of in-patient services was undecided although the trend is to avoid duplication.

Dr (later Professor) Grahame was Honorary Medical Secretary of ARC. He retired from Guy's in 1995 but continued his long-term interest in hypermobility syndromes from University College Hospital in London, an interest he shared with Paul Beighton (South Africa) and Howard Bird (Leeds). (Beighton, Grahame and Bird, 1998)

Grahame believed that hypermobility was under-diagnosed by rheumatologists. It was a feature of a number of named congenital disorders of connective tissue. It also occurred in otherwise normal people based on what might be called 'second class collagenous tissue.' Joint hypermobiliy might direct young people into netball, dancing, gymnastics and music but at the same time exposed them to more injuries, leading to secondary osteoarthritis, distinguishable sometimes from that which occurred in those without hypermobility.

The 'second class collagen' concept suggested an overlap with osteoporosis. Grahame found that as a group most hypermobile people had a bone mineral density in the lower part of the normal range. Studies showed a significant tendency to osteoporosis in the Ehlers-Danlos Syndrome.

King's College Hospital

George Frederick Still was the first Professor of Paediatrics at King's College Hospital in South London. When a medical registrar at the Great Ormond Street Hospital for Sick Children in 1897 he had written a paper 'On a form of chronic joint disease in children' that for a 60 years was to be known as Still's Disease. Before the war, Frank Cooksey of the Department of Physical Medicine had joined the committees and informal groups that were planning the 1943 inauguration of the British Association for Physical Medicine. Cooksey, like other consultants in Physical Medicine, was concerned with the rehabilitation of war casualties and was notable for his enthusiasm for civilian rehabilitation and occupational therapy. He was assisted by a remarkable woman occupational therapist, Gwendolyn McCaul. Between McCaul and Cooksey much of the 'rubbish' of occupational therapy training was eliminated. Cooksey initiated a common preliminary training for physiotherapists and occupational therapists. The rehabilitation department at King's College Hospital was famous for having part of a London bus and later a mock-up house for training in activities of daily living. It had a rehabilitation workshop run by a skilled craftsman, probably the first in a London teaching hospital and a forerunner of rehabilitation departments elsewhere. Cooksey was also interested in resettlement clinics but not in rheumatoid arthritis and used to pass all his rheumatology patients to colleagues. This did not deter him from explaining to a meeting of the Heberden Society at Hammersmith how to treat rheumatoid arthritis, an incident that prompted Professor Kellgren, with heavy irony, to stand up and thank Cooksey for his kind advice. Rheumatologists disliked the fact that Cooksey was Consultant Advisor to the Department of Health and Social Services in what the Department at the time grouped together as Physical Medicine and Rheumatology. Cooksey was not considered to be a rheumatologist by rheumatologists and they wanted someone else to advise the Department.

The first trained rheumatologist at King's was Dr Eric Hamilton, who qualified in 1952 from the Middlesex Hospital and recalled that there was at that time virtually no rheumatology teaching at student level there despite the link to the Arthur Stanley Institute. He did hear one lecture from Frank Howitt, an older physical medicine specialist, who had helped found both the Heberden Society and the British Association for Physical Medicine.

Hamilton was recruited to serve with the RAF Coastal Command and took part in the British North Greenland survey, surviving a plane crash. He worked at the Middlesex, Brompton and Hammersmith hospitals before becoming Registrar at Taplow. Jobs in rheumatology were scarce then so to improve his chances he sat and passed the Diploma of Physical Medicine. He became Senior Registrar at King's College Hospital and was promoted to Consultant in Rheumatology and Rehabilitation in 1962. Before Hamilton's arrival there was no single consultant in King's particularly interested in patients with arthritis, they were passed to whichever physician had available beds or out-patient space. When Cooksey retired in 1965 Dr John Goodwill who had been trained in rehabilitation medicine in Ann Arbor, USA replaced him. Dr. Philip Nichols and the author replaced him as consultant advisers to the Department of Health in rehabilitation and rheumatology respectively. Dr Hedley Berry joined Hamilton as second rheumatologist some years later.

In 1961 the Arthritis and Rheumatism Council endowed for ten years the 'Unit for Drug Action' at King's College Hospital under the direction of Dr MJH Smith. This explored the intermediary metabolism of salicylates and related anti-rheumatic drugs and took part in the ARC-sponsored International Symposium on Salicylates in 1962 under the chairmanship of Dr WSC Copeman.

Copeman as Chairman of the Executive Committee of ARC expressed irritation with this Unit and would have closed it if he could. He felt it was not sufficiently productive in terms of the hard won funds it absorbed. Others did not share this opinion.

At King's, Hamilton became a friend of Dr Roger Williams who was setting up his Liver Unit. After 1962, when Schumacher in the USA had drawn attention to the manifestations of this disease in the joints, Hamilton analysed the haemachromatosis patients attracted to the King's Liver Unit and published the first UK description of haemachromatosis arthropathy, drawing attention to the frequency and severity of the hip disease that it might cause. (Hamilton, Williams, Barlow et al.,1968). The association with the Liver Unit also led to publications on primary biliary cirrhosis, on the finger clubbing and osteoarthropathy that could complicate chronic liver disease, and on the hepatic changes that might be found in rheumatoid arthritis.

King's College Hospital had always, compared to the other teaching hospitals, suffered from a shortage of beds. Financial cutbacks could make the admission of arthritis patients with severe disease yet more difficult. It could be a problem for Professor DL Scott at Kings. He had been awarded a Medical Research Council grant of £994,000 to undertake the definitive study on the disease modifying drugs used for rheumatoid arthritis.

The Imperial College Schools of Science, Technology and Medicine.

St Mary's Hospital Medical School never built up a named Academic Department of Rheumatology and today it does not need one. For teaching purposes and research it is now part of a conglomerate of hospitals with academic departments in the west of London. One would have thought that St Mary's might have been an early entrant to rheumatology. After all, it had the laboratories where Sir Almoth Wright used to dispense autogenous vaccines for the proponents of focal sepsis in the Charterhouse Clinics. Professor Albert Neuberger, Heberden orator, was Principal of the Wright Fleming Institute from 1958 to 1962 and an expert on connective tissue chemistry, at that time the favoured science base for rheumatology research. But somehow it did not happen. Until 1948 St Mary's was an all-male medical school noted for its sporting prowess and perhaps rugby and rheumatology did not mix.

Dr Mary Carter was one of the first twelve women medical students to enter St Mary's (second Intake). At that time there were two physical medicine doctors, Drs Woodhouse and Hiscock, running a department for internal hospital referral only. Carter qualified in 1954 and after junior appointments at St Mary's transferred to Taplow as Registrar, later as Empire Rheumatism Council Research Fellow in the Special Unit for Juvenile (and by then adult) Rheumatism over a six year period. She returned to St Mary's in 1962 as Senior Registrar in general medicine. As the only physician in the hospital with full rheumatology training she was allowed to receive internal referrals. These rapidly extended to out-patients under the nominal aegis of her consultant. From 1965 to 1970 she was given consultant status and worked with endocrinologist Prof. VHT James, doing clinical research on the effects of corticotrophin and corticosteroids in rheumatic diseases. She was supported jointly by the Arthritis and Rheumatism Council and the Edgar Lawley Trust. In 1971 she was appointed as a National Health Service consultant and Honorary Clinical Senior lecturer, the first woman clinical consultant in the hospital and the first to sit on the Medical Committee of the Hospital. Soon after this the hospital was given a government grant of £150,000 for her to develop an inpatient rehabilitation department at the St Mary's, Harrow Road, hospital which would include a back pain service. It was closed two years after it was opened as a result of Area Health Authority cuts. Her efforts to prevent this resulted in a year stay of execution but received little support from consultant colleagues.

In 1974 Dr Martin Seifert who had trained in rheumatology at St Thomas's Hospital and at the Colorado Springs Hospital in Denver joined her. This was also a NHS appointment with an honorary teaching contract. Students spoke favourably about the quality of instruction in rheumatology despite the absence of a formal academic department,

Paediatric rheumatology problems at St Mary's were referred to Prof. Woo at Great Ormond Street Hospital for Sick Children. Surgical rheumatology was catered for by a hand surgeon and by another who dealt mainly with shoulders and elbows. There was a combined upper limb clinic with rheumatology. Another surgeon specialised in back problems and all took a share in the surgery of hips and knees. No one surgeon was particularly interested in foot problems but a podiatrist was in attendance if needed.

Dr Carter retired in1991 and was replaced by Dr Richard Rees who had trained in rheumatology at the Charing Cross hospital.

Dr Carter moved into the new Imperial College preclinical medical school in the department of medical and biological systems, working with the Professorial Head of Department and two bioengineer/physicist colleagues on the Knee Arthritis Project. The group aimed to develop a design sequence for nuclear magnetic resonance imaging of knees that could be of importance for when it will be possible to treat knee damage with intra-articular seeding of cultured cartilage.

The Charing Cross Hospital

The original *Charing Cross Hospital and Medical School* was small and situated in central London overlooking the Charing Cross Railway terminus near Trafalgar Square. It neither had space for preclinical studies nor room to expand. It was moved to the Fulham Palace Road in West London in 1967.

When the West London Hospital in Hammersmith was merged with the new Charing Cross Hospital the Kennedy Institute of Rheumatology became in effect the rheumatism research wing of The Charing Cross hospital. The Kennedy Institute had been built in Bute Street adjacent to the West London Hospital and stayed there until 1994 when it moved into the vacated Sunley buildings on Fulham Palace Road site. Dr Tom Scott, previously at Hammersmith Hospital, was appointed as consultant in medicine and rheumatology to the Charing Cross Hospital shortly before it moved to Fulham. After the move he became the Deputy Director of the Kennedy institute. Scott was for many year the Editor of the Annals of Rheumatic Diseases and the Editor of the later editions of Copeman's Textbook of the Rheumatic diseases. He was particularly interested in gout and will be remembered as the one who reversed the Hippocratic aphorism with the title 'A Eunuch takes the Gout'

Academic Rheumatology was represented by Professor R N Maini who later became Director of the Kennedy Institute. Under his direction the Institute achieved fame through demonstration that anti-Tumour Necrosis Factor-α could bring about remissions in rheumatoid arthritis, opening up a new avenue for therapeutics for this disease.

The Westminster Hospital was another small London medical school situated too near the centre of London at Dean Ryle street to be viable. When it closed its staff were moved into the new Westminster and Chelsea Hospital on the old St Stephen's Hospital site. This did not happen without opposition from those who worked there including Professor Derek Brewerton. They were concerned lest the history and traditions of the hospital would be lost. Westminster was notable as the hospital were Dr Frank Dudley Hart worked and taught and where he set up the first rheumatology service in a London teaching hospital.

In 1973 Drs Caffrey and James of the Westminster Hospital published their observation on an inherited predisposition to ankylosing spondylitis linked to the human leucocyte antigen, HLA B27. (Caffrey and James, 1973). The same observation was made at the time by a team in Los Angeles. The clinical staff were quick to realise and explore the importance of the discovery (Brewerton et al., 1973)

The medical schools of the Westminster and Charing Cross hospitals were merged in 1990. When in1992 health services were re-organised in the west of London, the medical schools of St Mary's, the Chelsea and Westminster and the Charing Cross hospitals were joined with the postgraduate medical schools at Hammersmith and Northwick Park to form the Imperial College of Science, Technology and Medicine.

Today registrars and trainees in rheumatology in St Mary's, for example, can rotate around appropriate academic departments in other hospitals. Individualised training paths can be offered to them. Under the new Directorate at St Mary's rheumatology is linked to cardiology for undergraduate training. Regular rheumatology teaching sessions are held in the associated hospitals and attendance is mandatory for junior staff.

The Royal Hospitals

The Royal London Hospital could have claimed in 1936 to be the earliest teaching hospital to have a rheumatism service when Sir Robert Stanton Woods' Department of Physical Medicine was allocated six beds for the 'Investigation and treatment of patients with rheumatic diseases'. It also had a strong neurological department under the direction of Sir Russell Brain that was interested in the spine. His assistant in 1953, Dr Marcia Wilkinson, received support from the Oliver Bird Fund for her pioneering anatomical and histological studies on cervical disc degeneration and the clinical syndromes arising therefrom.

Two rheumatologists from the hospital were to make significant contributions to the leadership of the Arthritis and Rheumatism Council (ARC) during its increasing importance to UK rheumatology.

Dr Michael Mason took over the office of Chairman of the Executive committee of the ARC when Copeman died. Later, when Mason died Dr.Colin Barnes succeeded him. Dr Gareth Jones, when a lay member of the Executive Committee of the ARC, was particularly grateful to Mason for his ability to explain in non-technical language 'what was going on'. Mason led in shedding the label 'Physical Medicine' which dogged for too long those who wished to study and treat patients with rheumatic disease along scientific lines.

Mason was born in 1917, qualifying during the war from St Bartholomew's hospital. After his war and post war service with the Royal Air Force he became Senior Registrar to Drs Will Copeman and Oswald Savage and in 1955 was promoted to Consultant in Physical Medicine at the London Hospital, working alongside Dr Will Tegner, the successor to Sir Stanton Woods. It was a cordial relationship and in 1960 they renamed their department Physical Medicine and Rheumatology. From the combined department came a number of scientific papers. There were controlled trials of unorthodox treatments such as faith healing and osteopathy, with largely negative results. On a more serious level a study of azathioprine in rheumatoid arthritis broke new ground by proving that it had an important corticosteroid-sparing effect. A study of men with seronegative arthritis or ankylosing spondylitis showed an increased incidence of prostatitis as judged by inflammatory cells in routine prostatic smears, thus broadening the concept of Reiter's syndrome.

Copeman, pursuing a vision of an academic rheumatology unit in every London teaching hospital, was active in getting the London Hospital authorities to agree to an ARC-funded Senior Lecturership that after five years was to be taken over by the Medical College. Dr Harry Currey was appointed in 1967.

Currey had been attached to the department of rheumatology under Professor Bywaters at Hammersmith Hospital. He had been trained in Cape Town but preferred to work in England. Dr Barry Vernon-Roberts (ARC-supported Senior Lecturer in Pathology), Mr. Michael Freeman, an orthopaedic surgeon working on the problems of prosthetic knee replacement, and Dr Currey jointly formed the London Hospital Bone and Joint Research Group. The Group had no common premises until 1976 when the ARC negotiated an arrangement with the Special Trustees of the London Hospital to build a laboratory block. The original concept of 'three bright young men' working together as a multi-disciplinary team had to change when Vernon-Roberts left for Australia. He was succeeded by Dr (now Prof.) Peter Revel who later moved to the Royal Free hospital. Drs John Van der Walt and Adam Coumbe maintain the interest and training in osteoarticular pathology.

The building came in handy when the Special Unit for Juvenile Rheumatism at Taplow closed and John Holborow, an MRC employee and later Professor, needed somewhere to continue his immunology progamme. Prof. Bywaters in his retirement also used it to study pathological specimens. It was the main base for Currey's successor in 1996, Professor David Blake, and his Inflammation Research Group team.

Currey was sequentially Reader, then Professor with a personal Chair that was later endowed by the ARC. He served 20 years, retiring in 1986. He died in 1998.

Dr Colin Greenhill Barnes was born in 1936 and qualified from the London Hospital in 1961. He was House Physician to Prof. Bywaters at Hammersmith and later Senior Registrar to Drs Mason and Tegner in the Department of Physical Medicine and Rheumatology, eventually succeeding Will Tegner on his retirement.

Barnes was Junior Honorary Medical Secretary of the ARC and he succeeded Mason as Chairman of the Executive and Finance Committee of ARC after Mason's untimely death in June 1977 while at a conference in San Francisco. During his career Barnes has been Consultant in rheumatology to the Notley Hospital and the St Luke's Hospital for the Clergy. He has also been President of the European and British Leagues against Rheumatism. He retired as chairman of the Executive and Finance Committee of ARC in 1993 but was recalled to take over again when his successor Prof. Verna Wright fell ill.

During Barnes' time the ARC adapted its constitution to conform to new Charity laws. From 29th of January 1998 the name was changed from the cumbersome 'Arthritis and Rheumatism Council For Research in Great Britain and the Commonwealth' to 'Arthritis Research Campaign', dropping the devalued word 'rheumatism' and at the same time retaining the initials by which it was known. A Board of Trustees rather than an executive committee now governs it.

Under the leadership of Mason and Barnes the ARC's policy was to endow personal Chairs during the working lifetime of the incumbent if there was a danger that the position might be lost on retirement. Fully endowed Chairs are now in place at Leeds, Birmingham, Bristol, Guy's, the Royal Free and the Royal London Hospitals and partly endowed Chairs at Edinburgh and Glasgow.

Barnes' special interest in rheumatology was Behçet's Disease. He set up a thriving Behçet's Disease Study Group that numbered 24 people from 17 different countries. The group had introduced an internationally agreed definition of the disease. There are many manifestations of Behçet's disease so the diagnosis depended on the presence of a required number of inclusion criteria and the absence of exclusion criteria. In 1998 Dr David Perry had the unwieldy title of 'Clinical Director of the Musculoskeletal Directorate (Rheumatology and Orthopaedics) of the Royal Hospitals National Health Service Trust' and Prof. Blake had moved to Bath.

St Bartholomew's Hospital.

The other partner in the Royal Hospitals Trust was St Bartholomew's

Hospital. St Bartholomew's, always known as Barts, was the oldest hospital in London and important to the history of modern rheumatology. No less than seven out of the twenty nine Presidents of the Heberden Society trained there as part of their careers, (Ernest Fletcher, Charles Heald, Sydney Twistington Higgs, Thomas Horder, George Kersley, Michael Mason, Oswald Savage,) and one Heberden Roundsman, (Wykeham Balme). while Professor Ronald Tunbridge, a Bart's alumnus, was a prime mover in setting up academic rheumatology in Leeds University. Other ex-Bart's academics that had made notable contributions to rheumatology included Professors Philip Wood, Derek Willoughby, Paul Dieppe and Paul Bacon and Dr Tony Thould. The consultant who in much of the early part of the last 50 years was in charge of rheumatology at St Bartholomew's was Dr Harold Wykeham Balme, a most modest man. Dr Will Copeman in his drive to establish academic rheumatology in every London teaching hospital was irked by the apparent lack of progress in Bart's.

Perhaps a comment by Dr Thould can cast light on the paradox. Wykeham Balme, he recalled, 'taught little but provided opportunities for learning'. Copeman tried to put pressure on Wykhame Balme to give the Heberden Round, the annual meeting of rheumatologists where one of their number demonstrates unusual or interesting patients he has treated. Eventually Balme capitulated, but Thould remembers that just before the event Balme was in tears regretting that in former years he 'had not done anything'. He was of course an excellent and percipient doctor but less than keen on adding to the literature explosion. Those who worked with him remember him with affection.

His colleague in rheumatology at the Hospital was Dr Ted Huskisson, also a Heberden Roundsman, who qualified in 1964 from the Westminster Hospital. Huskisson explored the interface between medical industry and academic rheumatology, with particular reference to clinical trials of new non-steroidal anti-rheumatic drugs. He pointed out that it was useful to have a variety available, as some patients would respond to one drug but not to another. With his mentor at the Westminster Hosital, Dr F D Hart, he wrote a book entitled 'All the Arthropathies'. He exposed 'Seatone', a preparation of the dried gonads of New Zealand green-lipped mussels, promoted world-wide as a cure for rheumatoid arthritis. He found it indistinguishable from powdered fishmeal in a controlled trial.

Huskisson helped found the peer-reviewed *European Journal of Inflammation,* a publication in which reports of clinical trials of anti-inflammatory drugs, not popular with rheumatology journals, could find a home. The journal inadvertently presented a loophole through which a drug company could gain publicity for its product without the usual scientific safeguards. The problem was exposed after a number of UK rheumatologists were taken by a sponsoring company on an elaborate junket to Venice and put up in style in a hotel to present or to listen to generally laudatory reports on the company's new drug indoprofen. The '*European Journal of Inflammation',* that published the proceedings of the conference as a supplement without peer review, came in for criticism when indoprofen had later to be withdrawn on grounds of safety and lack of efficacy. The conference was denounced as a corrupt 'freebie' and hospital authorities thenceforward looked twice at applications to attend anything similar.

Despite its age and traditions, St Bartholomew's seems destined to lesser roles. Already important bits have moved elsewhere. Professor DL Scott transferred to King's College hospital. The old hospital, sandwiched between London's financial district and a meat market, does not have a natural catchment area. People do not live there any more; they commute from the suburbs.

St George's Hospital

It was to the suburbs in Tooting that *St George's Hospital* and medical school moved in the 1970s, when the original prime site on the corner of Hyde Park became too small. This proved to be a smart move indeed. Clearly someone had studied a map of the distribution of teaching hospitals in London and seen that there was a sector of relative scarcity in the southwestern suburbs. Today St George's is the only medical school in London to have retained its independence.

When at Hyde Park Corner St George's was a small teaching hospital. Students enrolled there had to do their pre-clinical studies elsewhere. The move to Tooting began in the early eighties, departments transferring in phases first to the Grove hospital, previously an infectious disease hospital. Since then everything had expanded and the medical school had developed its own preclinical departments

The senior rheumatologist, Dr Felix Bruckner, qualified from the London Hospital in 1960 and was author of a study of adhesive capsulitis of the shoulder, published in the prestigious Quarterly Journal of Medicine in 1981. He was joined in 1976 by Dr David Jenkins. Jenkins was called up to do his National Service with the Army after the war and stayed on in the RAMC. He specialised in physical medicine and rehabilitation and was at one time seconded to Hammersmith Hospital and Taplow to gain experience in rheumatology with Drs Ansell and Bywaters. At St George's he was in charge of the (mainly neurological) rehabilitation services attached to the Atkinson Morley Hospital but continued as well in rheumatology until he retired.

At St George's Dr Tim Chambers was doing pioneering work on the basic biology of osteoporosis. There was also an Academic Rheumatology Unit within the Department of Immunology where Dr John Axford had a special interest in the oligosaccharide moiety of immunoglobulins. This had arisen out of the observation that abnormalities of bound galactose in immunoglobulin-G (IgG) occurred in rheumatoid arthritis and might be related to the chronicity of auto-immunity in that disease. Axford had qualified from University College and trained with Prof. Ivan Roit at the Bloomsbury Rheumatism Unit.

The Northern Hospitals Group. (Middlesex, University College and Royal Free hospitals)

The Middlesex Hospital was where Dr Will Copeman had his early consultant appointment. The British Red Cross Society's Clinic for Rheumatic Diseases at Peto Place, that played such a large part in the pre-war days of rheumatology, was moved there when it was renamed the Arthur Stanley Institute and taken over by the National Health Service. Middlesex Hospital was where Prof. Eric Bywaters trained and learnt his pathology at the Bland Sutton Institute and started work on the metabolism of articular cartilage. Later Prof. Keele did important work there on the chemistry of pain. A separate department of Immunology under Prof. Ivan Roitt gained international reputation for its work on autoimmune diseases. Some of the first follow-up studies on early rheumatoid arthritis were conducted there. Yet it is worth recalling that it was there that Dr Eric Hamilton when a student, and despite the link with the Arthur Stanley Institute, had virtually no undergraduate instruction in rheumatology. The senior rheumatologist in the twenty years post war was Dr AC ('Bill') Boyle who was not much interested in research. During his time a number of well-trained rheumatologists issued from his department. This point was emphasised in Dr DL Woolf's obituary of him 'He contributed much to the training of junior staff, emphasising clinical skills'.

In the 1980s the Middlessex Hospital merged with the *University College Hospital* to form the Bloomsbury hospitals. This added to rheumatology the specialised work of Prof. Dr David Isenberg on lupus and the work on muscles initiated by Professor Richard Edwards. Professor Edwards later transferred to the Chair of Medicine at Liverpool.[6] . Dr Pat Woo, when at the Hammersmith Hospital in 1994 became the first UK professor of paediatric rheumatology. She is now based at the University College, London whence she directs adolescent rheumatology at the Middlesex Hospital and paediatric rheumatology at the Great Ormond Street Hospital for Sick Children. (The history of paediatric rheumatology is considered further in Chapter 7).

The Arthritis Research Campaign had also designated and supported a Centre for Rheumatology at University College, London, (the academic wing of University College Hospital) under the direction of Prof. David Isenberg. Prof. Jonathan Edwards joined him. Edwards has suggested that rheumatoid arthritis resulted from a chance development of self-immortalising B-lymphocyte clones that secreted IgG-rheumatoid factor.

Expertise in basic science and immunology and the historically close links with the Royal National Orthopaedic Hospital, now at Stanmore, should ensure a balance of training and research at all levels.

The *Royal Free Hospital,* the third member of the group, was once a small hospital in the Gray's Inn Road taking only women medical students. Dr AT Richardson, who trained with Philipe Bauwens at St Thomas's, was physical medicine consultant there but electrodiagnosis was probably his chief field of interest. Like St George's the Royal Free found itself cramped for space. It moved out to Hampstead, but not far enough to escape being netted in with the Bloomsbury hospitals to form the Northern Group in the London Teaching Hospitals reorganisation. Dr Carol Black, who had qualified from Bristol in 1970 and worked with Malcolm Jayson on mechanisms of fibrosis before moving to the West Middlesex Hospital, became the ARC Professor of Rheumatology at the Royal Free Hospital and a world authority on systemic sclerosis and Raynaud's phenomenon. She directs the National Scleroderma Service.

6 A physiotherapist in the Muscle Unit, Di Newham, rashly undertook to exercise to the point of severe muscle stiffness the following day and then to have a quadriceps muscle biopsy. The histology showed widespread muscle damage, strikingly reminiscent of dermatomyositis. The changes healed rapidly.

Chapter 4.

Development of Rheumatology in the Provincial Teaching Hospitals.

While rheumatology was spreading in London, teaching hospitals in the rest of the United Kingdom were not being left behind. But there were exceptions.

Teaching hospitals in England

Bristol

The Professor of Medicine in Bristol, the late Bruce Perry, will be remembered with respect and affection by many for his clinical expertise and for championing the restoration of Jenner's 'Temple of Vaccinia'. But the development of rheumatology in Bristol had to await his retirement.

Perry had been a founder member of the Empire Rheumatism Council and a member of the Heberden Society when rheumatic fever and rheumatic heart disease were rife. But he had little time for patients with chronic rheumatic diseases. They were looked after by a weekly visit from Bath by Dr George Kersley to Southmead Hospital (but not in the prestigious Bristol Royal Infirmary). Perry is on record as saying that beds for chronic rheumatic diseases merited no more than part of a general medical ward. 'We tried this, and it was awful' Dr John Cosh recalls, when reconstruction of the Royal National Hospital for Rheumatic Diseases forced a temporary move to a ward in a general hospital.

The Medical Research Council funded Rheumatism Research laboratory at Bath was wound up during that reconstruction and in compensation a Lecturer in Rheumatology appointment was organised, to be shared between Bath and Bristol. The first holder, Dr Donald Ward had worked on iron metabolism in rheumatoid arthritis before moving to Oswestry. His successor Dr Malcolm Jayson chose to spend most of his time at Bath, where the facilities were better and the atmosphere more congenial. He worked jointly on the morbid physiology of raised intra-articular pressure, the experimenters having their own knees catheterised and distended with fluid. In Bath he pioneered the use of the arthroscope in rheumatology.

In 1969 Jayson was promoted to Honorary Senior Lecturer (Consultant) at Bristol and took the opportunity to establish rheumatology beds and clinics in Bristol, at first in the Bristol Homeopathic Hospital, later in the Royal Infirmary. Whereas Prof. Perry had been antagonistic, his successor, Prof. Alan Read was supportive, at least initially. Dr Richard Jacoby assisted as Lecturer and Dr Carol Black as Research Fellow. Dr Roger Bucknall studied the immune response in rheumatoid arthritis, and later became Consultant at the Royal Liverpool Infirmary.

Jayson worked with physicist Prof. Jito Shah on the crimp structure of collagen showing that collagen fibres had a degree of elasticity. With Alan Bailey of the Agricultural Research Council Meat Research Institute he studied factors affecting the cross-linkage and hence the 'toughness' (in meat terms) of collagenous structures. With Carol Black he used this knowledge to study systemic sclerosis and the skin thickening caused by vinyl chloride exposure. Assisted by Dr Mike Martin and others, he built up Bristol undergraduate rheumatology teaching that had previously relied upon visits to Bath. Meanwhile, Dr Paul Bacon who succeeded Kersley took over the Southmead commitment. When in 1978 Jayson became Professor of Rheumatology at Manchester he left behind a rapidly developing Department of Rheumatology which included a combined rheumatology/orthopaedic clinic with Mr Tony Ratliff, who had trained with John Charnley in Wrightington Hospital. A combined ophthalmological clinic enabled early studies of scleritis, scleromalacia and the corneal melt syndrome.

His successor Dr Paul Dieppe found Prof. Read by this time somewhat indifferent to rheumatology and he had a struggle to build up his research facilities. The Senior Registrar/Lecturer post alternating between Bristol and Bath continued and holders (and where they went to) included Charles Hutton (Plymouth), Diana McFarlane, (Guy's), Tony Woolf (Truro) and Michael Doherty (Nottingham). Giles Campion went to medical industry in the United States. When Paul Bacon accepted the Chair of Rheumatology in Birmingham, the Southmead/Bath link terminated. Dieppe also ended the shared lecturer arrangement with Bath although mutual visits continued. Dieppe saw these changes as necessary in order to have control over the planning and development of rheumatology in Bristol.

Bacon's successor at Southmead, Dr Peter Hollingsworth took over paediatric rheumatology.

The main thrust of Dieppe's research had been in osteoarthritis and chondrocalcinosis but other interesting studies included the arthritis caused by the parvovirus. The Blood Transfusion Centre in Southmead enabled co-operation with Dr Tim Wallington and others in immunocytology.

The chief of orthopaedic surgery, Mr Michael McCormack, was also supportive. Curiously Prof. Read, a gastroenterologist, did not take advantage of the active rheumatology unit within his department and the opportunities for shared interest, such as the association of chronic inflammatory bowel diseases and arthritis or the effects of anti-rheumatic drugs on the gastrointestinal tract. Dieppe had another struggle to get protected rheumatology beds, and eventually these became available in the Bristol Eye Hospital.

The Department of Pathology under Professor Epstein was not particularly interested in the rheumatic diseases but Dieppe had excellent co-operation from Dr Ian Watt whom he regarded as the 'best osteoarticular radiologist in the world'. Their technetium studies proved beyond doubt that osteoarthritis began as an inflammatory disease, and was not just 'wear and tear' as suggested by the previous name osteoarthrosis.

Dieppe, as Arthritis and Rheumatism Council Professor of Rheumatology, not only built up a strong department but also was able to do outreach clinics at Weston super Mare, where a new district general hospital had had no rheumatology presence. With Dr John Klippel of Bethesda he edited a major, heavyweight (*It weighed five and a half kilograms)* international textbook of rheumatology. Notoriety of an unwelcome sort came when he was in a civil aeroplane that landed in Kuwait just at the onset of the

Iraqi invasion and he was taken prisoner. He was in danger of being used as a human shield when the Allied forces began bombing. He was eventually released without physical harm.

Towards the end of his tenure, Dieppe became increasingly involved with administration and in 1995 resigned to become Dean, later working for the Senate but he retained a weekly presence in rheumatology with his colleague Dr John Kirwan. Dieppe's extensive work has made him a world expert on osteoarthritis. Dr, now Prof., Michael Doherty in Nottingham has picked up that particular baton.

Stoke Mandeville

Two of the early Edinburgh alumni, Alan Hill and Alastair Mowat, became consultants in the Oxford hospital region.

Dr Alan Hill was relatively well provided for when he moved from Edinburgh to Stoke Mandeville Hospital near Aylesbury. This hospital had been an Emergency Medical Service hospital during the war and had been recently changed to a general hospital to include a rheumatism unit. There were also spinal injuries and plastic surgery units that had originally been under the direction of the Ministry of Pensions. The rheumatism unit had 12 beds and benefited from the excellent occupational therapy, physiotherapy and hydrotherapy services provided for the spinally injured.

A Medical Research Council electromedical unit under Drs Bourdillon and Richie Russell was studying the blood brain barrier in multiple sclerosis and other neurological diseases. It added to the research interest in the hospital.

Hill found that a rise in C-reactive protein was a good indicator of the severity of rheumatoid arthritis but less so of systemic lupus. His study of early rheumatoid arthritis showed that patients who had positive blood tests for rheumatoid factor when first seen, or whose tests became positive in the first year of follow-up, had a worse prognosis than those whose tests remained negative at one year. His pathologist colleague Colin Tribe, who unfortunately died young, studied rectal biopsies in rheumatoid arthritis and showed that this was the method of choice for the early detection of amyloidosis.

With his colleague Virginia Camp, aided by the diligent co-ordinating powers of Dr Hugh Lyle of the drug company Dista, Hill was one of a large group who staged an exemplary multicentre trial of penicillamine in rheumatoid arthritis. This proved the effectiveness of this drug as a second-line or remission-inducing agent in this disease. (Andrews and others, 1973). As a result penicillamine began to replace gold or anti-malarial treatments and has outranked it in a five-year follow-up of disease modifying anti-rheumatic drugs conducted in South Wales (Jessop et al., 1998).

Oxford

Dr Alastair Mowat also took part in the original study of penicillamine. Mowat was appointed as Consultant Rheumatologist in the Nuffield Orthopaedic Hospital in Oxford where his surgical colleagues were pioneering reparative and salvage operations in arthritis. As such he was well placed to write the chapter on the surgical treatment of rheumatoid arthritis in the Fifth Edition of Copeman's Textbook of the Rheumatic Diseases. His particular laboratory research interest was in the factors that affected the chemotaxis of polymorphonuclear cells in rheumatoid arthritis, his clinical research interests included polymyalgia rheumatica. This last interest he handed on in turn to his senior registrar Brian Hazleman. Sheffield rheumatologists John Moll and Michael Snaith trained at Oxford, as did Paul Wordsworth of the Welcome Trust for Human Genetics. The latter is scanning the human genome for additional markers for an inherited predisposition to ankylosing spondylitis and related inflammatory rheumatic diseases.

Cambridge

Brian Hazleman was appointed Consultant Rheumatologist to Addenbrooke's hospital in Cambridge in 1973. Prior to his appointment Cambridge rheumatology patients were looked after by Dr Chalmers, a general physician, by Dr Fell, a physical medicine specialist and by Dr Randall a rehabilitationist previously at the Hospital for Nervous Diseases at Queen's Square in London.

On his appointment, which was 'received with some apathy' by the then Addenbrooke's general physicians, he was allotted four beds at Newmarket Hospital and out-patient clinics at King's Lynn, Saffron Walden and Ely hospitals. This was at a time when the new Addenbrooke's was still being commissioned and many of its staff did not think that a university style medical school could or should develop in Cambridge. Sir Lionel Whitby, the first Heberden Roundsman, had said that the population served by Addenbrooke's was relatively small and so scattered that sufficient material for teaching would not be available. Nevertheless, a clinical school planning committee was founded in 1970 and the first clinical students were admitted in 1976.

When Newmarket Hospital closed in 1992, Hazleman was allocated a 19-bedded ward at Addenbrooke's.

For a long time he had no senior registrar. Those that trained with him as registrars and who are now consultants include Valerie Kyle (Southmead, Bristol), Richard Watts (Ipswich), Jill Pountain at Huntingdon, Di Bulgen at Chester and Alan Binder at the Lister hospital. There were also a number of trainees from Australasia and Europe.

Over the past 10 years he and Dr Jumbo Jenner (rehabilitation) were joined as consultant colleagues by Dr Adrian Crisp who had a special interest in osteoporosis and by Prof. John Hill Gaston, from Prof. Paul Bacon's unit in Birmingham, with a special interest in immunology. The scientific ambience was greatly strengthened when Prof. Keith Peters, who has been supportive of rheumatology, moved to Cambridge from the Royal Postgraduate Medical School in Hammersmith.

Hazleman traced his interest in soft tissue rheumatism and shoulder problems to Philip Nichols and in polymyalgia rheumatica to Alastair Mowat both at the Nuffield Orthopaedic Hospital in Oxford.

By 1999 the Cambridge rheumatology service had a 19-bedded dedicated rheumatology ward staffed by 16 nurses and two specialist nursing sisters. An occupational therapist and two physiotherapists were attached to the unit. There were two specialist registrars, a senior house officer and a house physician.

The rheumatology unit also benefited from advice from Prof. R Coombes as head of Immunology and his work on the initiation of arthritis. Advice was also available from the Dunn School of Nutrition (Dr. Kodicek with his interest in vitamin D), and from Drs Juliet Compston and Jonathan Reeve who combined with Dr Adrian Crisp to run the osteoporosis service.

The proximity of the Strangeways laboratories, which when under John Dingle's leadership worked on the bone and joint tissue problems, had been important to Cambridge rheumatology. In 1950-60 Dingle had been at the Royal National Hospital for Rheumatic Diseases in Bath in the 'Oxford and Southwest Rheumatism Research Laboratories' working on the metabolism of synovial tissue in rheumatoid arthritis. A Mr. Strangeways Pigg-Strangeways had originally set up the Strangeways Laboratory as a private venture in 1912 and had decided that the laboratory should concentrate on rheumatoid arthritis. In one experiment he paid a tramp to sleep three nights in the boggy fens to test the theory that rheumatoid arthritis was caused by damp and mist.

In 1924 Honor Fell, then aged 24, took over and the research veered towards developmental biology and the effects of Vitamin A on cultured embryonic cartilage. When Dingle joined he developed a method to culture adult cartilage. In 1970 Dingle became Director when Honor Fell retired but asked her to return to work. She did so until she died in 1988.

Under Dingle's leadership Strangeways built up an increasing reputation and most of its work was relevant to basic problems of bone and joint tissues, particularly cartilage. There were studies on metalloproteinases and their inhibitors and the discovery of 'catabolin' which turned out to be the same as Interleukin–1. Work was done on micro-encapsulation of steroids for intra-articular use. The Strangeways staff studied Bone Morphogenetic Protein, subsequently known to be a family of proteins that acted as attractants to osteocytes and which could form structured bone in vivo. Bone Morphogenetic Proteins were coming into commercial use for the repair of tooth to alveolar margin adhesion in gingivitis and their possibilities for osteoporosis were being explored. The staff numbers grew to 120 workers. Brian Hazleman was an honorary member.

In 1993 after Dingle retired the then Chairman (who was unwell but did not realise it) took personal charge of the laboratory. No new Director was appointed. The staff numbers fell from 120 to 20 in nine months as they were 'head-hunted' for other laboratories. The Chairman died six months later but the damage had been done. 'A great loss to rheumatology research. But numbers are now being built up again.' Strangeways has changed its focus and is now run by the Clinical Research Council

When Hazleman in 1998 succeeded Prof. Roger Sturrock as President of the British Society for Rheumatology he was considering how he could improve and extend rheumatology services during his tenure. There would be support for the combined Arthritis and Rheumatism Council / British Society for Rheumatology clinical trials initiative. This it was hoped would go some way to redress the perceived bias of ARC funding towards laboratory research. He saw the need to emphasise rheumatology care for the problems of sufferers from back, neck, shoulder and foot problems and to extend interest into sports medicine.

Leeds

In the early 1930s some confidence was returning to UK business after the dark days of the recession. Initiatives in London were striving to rebuild a national thrust against the chronic rheumatic diseases and Leeds University did not wish to be left out of those who would undertake the research. There were discussions with those physicians who also worked in Harrogate as to where this might best take place. In the event the University did not have the money while Harrogate did, thanks to an appeal headed by a local philanthropist, Lord Harewood. (Cantor, 1988). £10,000 was raised and a laboratory built. Pathologist Dr Douglas Collins was installed in 1934. He became the first such to specialise in the morbid anatomy of bone and joint disease in the UK, publishing a paper in the first volume of the *Annals of Rheumatic Diseases*, (1939). The importance of Harrogate was strengthened by its wartime role in rehabilitating military casualties. After the war under the influence of Professor Ronald Tunbridge, further efforts were made to establish rheumatology in Leeds hampered, according to Tunbridge, by opposition from Professor Stanley Hartfall. Hartfall had been Professor of Therapeutics in Leeds before the war. At that time he had a wide range of interests in medicine. Hartfall's personal Chair was changed to Professorship of Clinical Medicine in 1948, and after that he took a particular interest in rheumatology and was an early enthusiast for gold therapy for rheumatoid arthritis, incidentally a major contributor to his private practice. Meanwhile the dominance of Harrogate was being eroded. In part this was because Sir Stanley Davidson, then Professor of Medicine at Edinburgh, wearing his clinical pharmacology hat, had rubbished the spa facilities when he was commissioned to report on them for the Harrogate Borough Council after the war, (H.Bird). In part it was financial. 1949 saw the devaluation of the pound. Funding either from charitable or Council sources became less generous.

Trainees of the late Professor Verna Wright could, if they were so minded, trace their rheumatological lineage back to Ian Duthie and Edinburgh, as Wright was Alan Hill's first senior House Officer at Stoke Mandeville and Alan Hill had trained with Duthie. It was at Stoke Mandeville that Wright first began studying psoriatic arthritis. Wright became research assistant to Stanley Hartfall in 1956 and succeeded him on the latter's retirement in 1964. Wright rejuvenated Leeds' contribution to the fight against chronic rheumatic diseases.

Wright was born in Devonport in 1928, educated in Bedford, and obtained a State scholarship to Liverpool University to study veterinary medicine. He switched to human medicine and qualified in 1953. He spent a year in Johns Hopkins University on a fellowship and worked on biomechanics before returning to Leeds. Wright was awarded a personal Chair in 1970, later endowed by the Arthritis and Rheumatism Council.

Dr John Moll recounted the early and happy days of his postgraduate rheumatology training at Leeds after he joined Wright in 1969. Wright had chosen to concentrate on the spondylarthropathies, the word he had invented to cover the group of diseases associated with inflammatory polyarthritis and spondylitis but in which circulating rheumatoid factor was absent.

The work started with Dr Ian Macrea's survey of families with ulcerative colitis and arthritis. Moll undertook a family study of psoriatic arthritis. Dr Ian Haslock followed this with a similar study of Crohn's disease. Dr (now Professor) Ann Chamberlain's survey of Behçet's Disease followed and helped consolidate the concept of 'spondylarthropathies' at a time when knowledge of the inherited predisposing factor HLA B27 was only just emerging.

Wright always insisted that any research or study be brought to a conclusion such as a paper read to a learned society, a publication, or a presentation for a doctoral thesis. Moll and Wright were co-authors of a book on the spondylarthropathies (*Seronegative Polyarthritis,* 1976) and Moll worked with Wright and Haslock to write a chapter on the topic in *Copeman's Textbook of the Rheumatic Diseases* 5th and 6th editions. Moll later edited and contributed to a textbook on Ankylosing Spondylitis, the first in the UK.

Dr Howard Bird, previously at Bath, was appointed as consultant to the Leeds General Infirmary in 1980. One part of the job was to look after the University-linked beds at the Royal Bath Hospital in Harrogate. He took over the laboratories that Dr Douglas Collins had once occupied and established a pharmacology and clinical trials unit there. This was sponsored by drug manufacturers Roche but funding from that source ceased in 1993 when the company decided to withdraw from research into rheumatic diseases-related drugs. The writing was by then on the wall for the Royal Bath Hospital, the Harrogate Hospital Trust having weighed it in the funding balance and found it wanting. Conversely the change to Trust status gave Leeds the opportunity it had long hoped for- to bring all its rheumatology services within the city. Bird was given extensive new facilities for his clinical pharmacology unit at Chapel Allerton Hospital where he was appointed to the Chair in Developmental Pharmacological Rheumatology. He continued with his interest in the damage and disabilities arising out of sports and performing arts injuries and was also exploring the bone and joint problems of the hypermobility syndromes.

Another strand of the Leeds research under the direction of Wright was his association with medical engineering through Prof. Duncan Dowson and Dr Tony Unsworth. This included work on the stiffness of joints and also on the mechanical properties of cartilage, bones and ligaments. Wright and Dowson contributed a paper on the tribology of surfaces in motion in the book edited by MIV Jayson entitled 'Total Hip Replacement Arthroplasty'. One product of the bioengineering research was the 'Leeds ligament', the work of Dr Bahaa B Seedhom, used to mend badly torn ankle collateral ligaments, usually the result of skiing accidents and under development for replacement of the cruciate ligaments in the knee. Dr Chris Murray-Leslie, rheumatologist in Derby and himself a skydiver, inspired a comparative study of injuries to sporting and military parachutists.

Wright widened the concept of rheumatology in other directions. Dr Anne Chamberlain was in 1988 appointed as Charterhouse Professor of Rheumatological Rehabilitation. She has expanded her department with grants from European and Department of Health sources to 24 staff including three who were medically qualified.

They covered limb fitting, 'Possum' supply and servicing, and the assessment of severity of disability and consequent special needs. Her department is concerned with the rehabilitation of all patients with chronic diseases, not exclusively rheumatic diseases.

Surgical rheumatology in Leeds had been built up in co-operation with the Professor of Orthopaedic Surgery, Robert Dickson, and similar arrangements have been made for skin problems and paediatric rheumatology.

Numerous trainees had passed through Wright's department. Professor Bird had spent two weeks with Professor Philip Wood at the Arthritis and Rheumatism Council Unit for Epidemiological Research after leaving Bath. It was Wood's studies of the inequality of health care provision for the rheumatic diseases that lead Wright and Bird to promote the appointment of rheumatologists throughout the Yorkshire Region. As a result there were 24, at least one in every major district general hospital, a veritable explosion over the last 15 years with most of the new appointments since 1994.

This touched on a general problem that was beginning to affect provincial training centres for rheumatologists such as Bath, Leeds and Manchester. Leeds was no longer the first port of call for Yorkshire patients since they had a service in their local hospital. To retain its usefulness for patients other than the inhabitants of Leeds the 'Mother centre' had to diversify.

When Wright retired as Professor of Rheumatology in 1993 he was replaced by Prof. Paul Emery from Prof. Paul Bacon's service in Birmingham. Emery set up a study of early rheumatoid arthritis and the factors that indicated prognosis. This included a Region-wide standardised assessment of patients who presented with early arthritis. He investigated an array of modern imaging techniques and other tests and established that these could be used to predict the likelihood of poor outcome, and hence the justification for the use of stronger treatments for those most at risk of severe disease.

Professor Wright took over the Chairmanship of the Executive Committee of the Arthritis and Rheumatism Council following the retirement of Dr Colin Barnes. Wright developed cancer of the prostate from which he died on January 31st 1998 at the age of 69. He has left a considerable mark on UK rheumatology. From interviews with his colleagues of the early days one can build up a pen portrait.

Wright was very efficient and economical with his time, taking his personal tape recorder with him and dictating letters while in the car. He even continued dictating whilst awaiting rescue after his car had been involved in an accident. He nevertheless always managed to leave work at 5 PM, (but on Wednesdays he would have started at 7.30 am for his weekly research meeting.) He was good at delegation. If he put his trust in someone he would back what was done in his name. (Once when a letter had to be written to the Regional Board, he delegated the job of composing the letter to Ian Haslock and signed it without reading it). He was also egalitarian. The team would meet for coffee in the morning. Visitors found it strange that they would be introduced first to Mrs Proctor, the cleaner, the most senior woman present, then the other women, lastly the men, an example of old-fashioned courtesy. Religion was at the core of his life. John Moll recalls that as a boy of 13, walking to school in Leeds, he would cross to the other side of the road to avoid a young evangelist who had the embarrassing habit of pulling a listener out of the audience and questioning him about his beliefs. He did not then know that the evangelist was to be his boss. Wright always carried a bible with him in his pocket and used it to check up on biblical references. Tuesday lunchtimes he would preach on the steps of Leeds Town Hall. But he did not bring his religion into the day-to-day dealings with other people in the hospital nor try to convert them. Haslock recalled that he and Wright were known as 'Sin and Salvation'.

Sheffield

In 1911 the Medico-Mechanical Institute provided the first service akin to rheumatology and rehabilitation in Sheffield. The first Medical Director was Dr RG Abercrombie, who was also styled 'Physician in Orthopaedic Disorders'. The Institute was primarily an out-patient service, which included treatments for industrial injuries and, in its early years, expanded to cover the treatment for First World War wounded.

The first funding for the service came from Mr W Edgar Allen, a steel magnate in poor health. He set up the Institute out of his own funds and paid the running costs for the first three years. The establishment was later named after him, first as the Edgar Allen Institute and ultimately as the Edgar Allen Physical Treatment Centre. The Institute was situated in central Sheffield in Gell Street. Edgar Allen imported from Sweden a complete set of Zander treatments based on various mechanical and electrical devices. The Institute and other health services in Sheffield were later funded by Sheffield's innovative 'Penny in the Pound' scheme, whereby 1d per £1 was contributed by the people of the city from weekly wages and salaries. The system was to be adapted in other cities and in the pre-National Health Service era provided useful funding for better hospital services.

As early as 1920 there had been moves appealing to Yorkshire's local patriotism to set up a Yorkshire-wide fund for supporting rheumatism treatment and research. This was seen to involve moving the centre of such efforts to Leeds and its university. Despite a number of discussions and apparent agreement, the efforts always foundered on Leeds-Sheffield rivalry. Sheffield, which has been described as the biggest village in England, was proud of its Edgar Allen Physical Treatment Centre, probably the first in the country outside London and was wary of anything that might change it. After all, it was the working man in Sheffield who contributed to 'his' treatment centre through the 'Penny in the Pound'.

A Yorkshire wide scheme, suggested by the fund raiser BT Clegg in Leeds would inevitably be seeking major money from a few rich philanthropists. However, when the National Health Service in 1948 took over the Centre these rivalries ceased to be relevant.

Dr Harry West from Bristol was the first director of rheumatology services and research in Sheffield after the National Health Service had been set up. West had run a mission hospital in Jordan before the Second World War and during that war had served in the Royal Army Medical Corps with the Arab Legion and the

Transjordan Frontier Force. After being demobilised he set up the student health service in Bristol and took over Professor Bruce Perry's clinic for ankylosing spondylitis. There he noticed that ankylosing spondylitis seemed to run in families. He contacted all the relatives of his patients and investigated those who had symptoms of ankylosing spondylitis. His was the first UK publication on the familial aggregation of this disease. (West,1949)

West was appointed as Consultant to the United Sheffield Hospitals in charge of the Sheffield Centre for the Investigation and Treatment of the Rheumatic Diseases with beds at the Nether Edge Hospital and an out patient department at the Edgar Allen Centre. He served from 1950 to 1970. He accepted the job on condition that he would be given ample accommodation for a research unit and a chemical research laboratory in a Regional Board hospital. After three years he changed to working part-time with the National Health Service and part-time in the University, supported by a Nuffield Research Fellowship. Dr Reg Newns, who had been his registrar, became a consultant. When the 5-year Fellowship ended West became a member of the external staff of the Medical Research Council (MRC).

West had arrived in Sheffield at the time of the excitement about the discovery of the anti-inflammatory effects of cortisone and corticotrophin. It was thought that this was the area where the cause and cure of the inflammatory rheumatic diseases might be found. He acquired two steroid chemists and after two years their work provided the first chemical assay for the diagnosis of Addison's Disease. It also enabled physicians to control the dose of corticotrophin by its biological effectiveness. On the strength of this the Empire (later Arthritis and-) Rheumatism Council provided a 5-year fellowship for one of chemists (Konrad Norymberski). West's unit took part in the United Kingdom trials of cortisone and prednisolone in rheumatoid arthritis, starting in the early 1950s.

The laboratory research was funded from a local charity. A committee of professors that included Hans Krebs was set up and the Board of Governors provided money for staff. Dr West and Dr Norymberski parted company after five years, West considering that the biochemistry laboratory was insufficiently productive.

The Sheffield Centre embarked on a series of publications on the methodology of assay of cortisone and corticotrophin and on different regimes of treatment, some eighty publications in all. Along with the group under Dr Oswald Savage at the West London Hospital, he promoted the self-administration of corticotrophin by patients with rheumatoid arthritis. West's unit in its day had an excellent reputation and several young scientists who came to work there were subsequently awarded their Ph D's.

The main conclusion of the work on corticosteroids was that treatment of rheumatoid arthritis with prednisolone 5mg daily gave the best results in terms of disease control, did not cause adverse effects and reduced the incidence of new bone erosions.

That which stimulated interest in the relationship of the pituitary/adrenal axis to rheumatoid arthritis was the observation by Hench and others that rheumatoid arthritis would remit during pregnancy. Using the recently developed paper chromatography and gas chromatography methods West and his colleagues found the explanation. During pregnancy the degree of cortisol binding in the blood decreased, doubling the amount of active free hormone at the expense of inactive bound cortisol. This was later confirmed by assays in saliva, a pioneering use of saliva as a body fluid on which to mount diagnostic investigations, although common now in checking for illegal or recreational drugs. Their work was published in the *Journal of Endocrinology* and so did not receive much attention in the rheumatology community.

West retired at the age of 60, the rule for MRC employees. He was offered but declined a chair in Chemical Pathology. Newns retired in 1973 and moved to Norfolk. When West gave the Heberden Round in 1963, his subject was the long-term use of corticotrophin. He was President Elect of the Heberden Society in 1969 but his early retirement precluded his taking it up. He went to a 29-acre property at Widworthy, near Honiton, Devon, restoring it as a garden open to the public. He was also interested in writing on religious and philosophical themes. At the age of the 89 he is devoting himself to writing a book on natural philosophy, a synthesis, as it were, of known facts.

Thus West could look back to his achievements at Sheffield with some satisfaction. Some of his contemporaries, perhaps because he did not publish in the journals they read, were more sceptical. Prof. Bruce Perry, who visited West a few years after his appointment, reported (to John Cosh) that 'West lives in a kind of steroid fog'. Prof. Eric Bywaters remarked that the 'clinicians regarded him as a biochemist and the biochemists regarded him as a clinician'. When he was asked to recall the time when he served on the Research Committee of the Arthritis and Rheumatism Council West said that he always felt inhibited from applying for research grants or equipment for his own Unit. Did he set his face against any form of self-publicity? The impression he gave was that he felt that he could not seek ARC money lest he be accused of taking personal advantage of his position on the Research Committee. It may explain why some of his colleagues did not appreciate his work.

Dr West was succeeded in 1973 by Dr John Moll and Dr Newns was succeeded by Dr Rod Amos. Dr Sami Derini, who was a Registrar in the department from the early West-Newns days, was appointed Associate Specialist. Further departmental changes have included the succession of Dr John Titcombe, (Consultant in Physical Medicine), by Dr John Winfield, (Consultant in Rheumatology and Rehabilitation), and the appointment of Dr Deborah Bax as Consultant Rheumatologist on the retirement of Dr Derini. Including the Honorary Consultant Rheumatologist, Dr Snaith, the Department now has six consultants with the recent appointment of Dr Mohammed Akil. The rheumatology service at Nether Edge Hospital originally had 39 beds, but the number was reduced to 21 beds with the transfer to the Royal Hallamshire Hospital in June 1997.

After obtaining a PhD in medical communication, John Moll collaborated over some years in studies directed by Dr John Lawrence of the ARC Epidemiology Unit based at Manchester. The publications arising from this work concerned the genetics of ankylosing spondylitis and other spondylitic disorders.

Dr Amos and Dr Betty Priestley provided Paediatric rheumatology in Sheffield until her retirement. The service for osteoporosis and bone diseases was provided at the Northern General Hospital under the direction of Professor Richard

Eastell, with assistance from Dr. Bax. Orthopaedic surgery in Sheffield had always been strong. There were then 15 orthopaedic surgeons in Sheffield. Hip surgery was offered widely and there was considerable expertise in the surgery of other joints. Mr John Getty who has collaborated with the rheumatologists in combined orthopaedic-rheumatology clinics, preferred knee and other lower limb surgery and, with neurosurgical collaboration, had covered spinal work. Mr David Stanley provided an upper limb joint surgery service. Plastic surgeons Mr Bob Page and Mr Gavin Miller shared the hand reconstruction work.

Sheffield boasted three Professorial Chairs in bone medicine (occupied by Professors Graham Russell, John Kanis and Richard Eastell) and two in orthopaedics but none in rheumatology. Dr Barbara Ansell in 1987 when on a visit to Sheffield as Sir Ernest Finch Visiting Lecturer suggested that Sheffield should apply for an ARC-funded Lecturer post, with a view to taking on a younger person and bringing him or her on 'in house'. Her recommendation was based on the research achievements in rheumatology and the need to relieve the NHS staff of their increasing teaching commitments. It was not until 1991 that the go-ahead was received. It was decided that the new post should be at Senior Lecturer level. Dr M L Snaith, previously consultant rheumatologist at the Bloomsbury District Health Authority and President of the British Society for Rheumatology was appointed.

Moll was considering retiring early to expand his publishing and artistic interests. He was the author of several books (10 rheumatology, 3 medical history/portraitures, including his personally illustrated History of the Heberden Society'). He was founding editor of three journals. He planned to give more time to his latest publishing venture, *The Journal of Medical Biography*. His latest work was an edition of bronze commemorative medallions for the Royal Society of Medicine, the first of which was recently presented to the Princess Royal on the occasion of her Honorary Fellowship and Special Lecture.

Birmingham

Birmingham, the second city of the United Kingdom, together with the surrounding Black Country, houses about three and a half million people. In the 1950s it was relatively depleted of rheumatology expertise. There were three physicians who did this as part of their general medical work. One was Dr Clifford Hawkins who was also a gastroenterologist. In the Dudley Road Hospital Dr Ghillespie ran a rheumatology clinic as well as a diabetic clinic. Dr Marshall Phillip at Selly Oak hospital also saw rheumatism patients. There were a few Physicians in charge of Departments of Physical Medicine but they lacked access to beds. Patients seriously ill with rheumatoid arthritis were sent to one of the Spa hospitals, usually to Droitwich but sometimes to Bath or Buxton.

Hawkins approached the Governors of the Queen Elizabeth Hospital to put the case for a new Rheumatism Wing. The Chairman of the Governors was a Birmingham solicitor, Sir Evan Ag Norton, who was well connected with the leading Birmingham industrialists. Sir Evan raised funds from them to build the rheumatism wing. It was to be run by the Department of Experimental Pathology under Professor John Squire. Squire was due to leave Birmingham to advise on the development of the

Northwick Park Hospital, as a postgraduate medical school, so the job devolved on his Senior Lecturer, Dr Kenneth Walton.

Walton had been appointed as Lecturer in Pathology in 1948. He was later to become Professor of Experimental Pathology in 1966 and had a sustained interest in the scientific aspects of rheumatology. He retired in 1984.

Walton at short notice planned what was needed for the new Rheumatism Wing. Walton and Hawkins moved in but office space was left available for other Birmingham doctors with an interest in rheumatology. Walton recalls that his Dean telephoned one day to say the High Sheriff of Worcester was on the phone, complaining that he had not been informed about the fund-raising, 'He wants to give some money-it may be £50 or even £500. Would you ring him back?' Walton did, and was astonished to be told it was £50,000!

Dr Derek Felix-Davis, who had been away in 1961 as Visiting Professor in Buffalo, New York, was one of those who could have taken advantage of the new facilities for research. Sadly, he died young in a road traffic accident. Another was Dr Brian McConkey, also a 'physician with an interest' who had succeeded Dr Ghillespie in 1963.

Brian McConkey trained at Oxford, qualifying in 1946. He had been Senior Registrar at Cardiff working mainly at the Llandough Hospital. His consultant there was Dr Idris Jones, a physician who with McConkey was responsible for ward teaching of rheumatic diseases. He recalls that at his appointment committee for the Dudley Road job he was told that he was expected to look after the rheumatoid arthritis patients and collect their blood specimens but had to convey those specimens to the recently opened Rheumatic Diseases Wing for the research there. He viewed that particular instruction with some reserve but complied and turned it to his advantage by bringing for processing other specimens arising from his own research.

At Cardiff and later in Birmingham McConkey had worked on metabolic bone diseases with the late Paul Fourman and studied 'prednisolone purpura' with Prof. Sam Schuster showing that, as in senile purpura, it reflected the escape into atrophic skin of red cells that failed to undergo normal haemolysis. He suspected that the thin transparent skin on the backs of the hands of corticosteroid treated patients was an indicator of osteoporosis, both being associated with collagen atrophy. McConkey promoted the estimation of C-reactive protein in the assessment of the activity of the rheumatic diseases

Rheumatism research in Birmingham in the last 50 years had been supported by local and national funding agencies including the Arthritis Research Council and the Medical Research Council. The Oliver Bird Fund of the Nuffield Foundation had given £170,000 since 1948.

In 1950 £8,000 was awarded to Prof. Stacey for developing methods of analysing the chemistry of cartilage and connective tissue. In recent times Dr (now Prof.) DGI Scott and Prof. Paul Bacon received in 1984 £22,125 for work on vasculitis.

Walton was succeeded in 1981 by Paul Bacon as Professor of Rheumatology in the Queen Elizabeth Hospital with duties in Selly Oak Hospital and in

Highfield Hospital in Droitwich. Bacon had qualified at St Bartholomew's in 1963. He was a Senior Registrar at Bart's before being awarded a Fellowship in Rheumatology at the University of California with Carl Pearson. From 1971 to 1981 he was Consultant at the Royal National Hospital for Rheumatic Diseases in Bath before moving to Birmingham.

Prior to 1981 rheumatic patients needing long term care were sent to the Highfield Hospital in Droitwich where Dr John Popert had been appointed in 1966. Prof. Phillip Wood's analysis of consultant manpower showed that the West Midlands medical area had at that time the lowest number of rheumatologists per head of population and there was no stock of traditional Physical Medicine posts that might be converted to rheumatology.

Bacon's first task was to negotiate for Lecturer and Senior Lecturer posts with programmes that allowed for research as well as clinical duties. In the 18 years since his appointment the number of such posts has risen to five. Incumbents who have gone on to occupy professorial Chairs have been D. Blake (The London Hospital and Bath), J. Hill Gaston (Cambridge). P. Emery (Leeds), D.L. Scott (King's College), D.G.I. Scott, (Norfolk and Norwich) and T. Southwood, (Paediatric Rheumatology in Birmingham).

There were active support groups for patients with systemic lupus, scleroderma, Wegener's disease and vasculitis. Surgical rheumatology was another area where changes had to be made. In 1981 there were six orthopaedic surgeons, all generalists. (Bacon described himself as flabbergasted when he asked one orthopaedic surgeon to perform bilateral total hip replacement arthroplasty on a girl with ankylosis of both hips, and the surgeon did not seem to be able to absorb the idea.) Since then things had much improved.

Birmingham rheumatology had come a long way in a relatively short time. Bacon's Unit was particularly recognised for its contributions to the study of vasculitis in rheumatoid arthritis and Wegener's Syndrome and investigations into early arthritis in order to determine prognosis. But the imponderables of medicine were still important to him—"If patient satisfaction were an outcome measure of the effectiveness of a treatment we would still have the Spa hospitals".

Newcastle

Newcastle after the war was one among many centres for the reception of children with rheumatic fever and took part in the 1952 US-UK rheumatic fever, Cortisone, ACTH, Aspirin, treatment study.

The study and treatment of chronic rheumatic diseases can be said to have started with the appointment in 1955 of Dr Malcolm Thompson, born and bred a 'Geordie'. Thompson had trained in Duthie's unit in Edinburgh and at the Massachusetts General Hospital in Boston, after three years as Senior Registrar at the Newcastle General Hospital.

Thompson set up the rheumatology service in Newcastle but not without difficulty. The idea seems to have had a somewhat doubtful acceptance by the Professor of Medicine, Dr (later Sir) George Smart. Thompson had to make do at first with a 'closed' clinic, restricted to seeing patients referred from other consultants and he had no beds. He gradually overcame these hurdles and he was joined by Dr Molly Hall, who later moved to Caerphilly when her husband Reg Hall became Professor of Medicine in Cardiff.

When Thompson was invited to give the Heberden Round at the Royal Victoria Infirmary in 1964 the task had to be split between him and Sir George, the only instance of two people giving the Round.

Dr Ian Griffiths was appointed to the Freeman hospital and the Royal Victoria Infirmary in 1978 and joined by Dr Carson Dick from Glasgow as Reader the following year on funds donated by a local builder, William Leech. Griffiths gave the Heberden Round in 1990 and is Consultant Adviser in Rheumatology to the Chief Medical Officer in the Department of Health.

Malcolm Thompson retired in 1984 and was replaced by Dr Philip Plat. Thompson had been socially and politically conscious. He organised regular swimming sessions for his patients and bus tour holidays in Europe for those who were disabled. He was elected Alderman in 1967 and was awarded the MBE.

Dr David Walker was appointed to the Newcastle and North Tyne hospitals in 1988. Others who were part of the rheumatology team were Drs PR Crook and Helen Foster (who looked after paediatric rheumatology). Carson Dick, always a stimulating if somewhat flamboyant figure, died in 1994. Prof. Tim Cawston from Cambridge and the Strangeways Laboratories was appointed in 1995 as the first UK non-clinical Professor of Rheumatology. A combined musculoskeletal Unit was formed in 1984. (However, research on muscles was not part of the Unit's remit. That stayed with the neurologists following the tradition established by Sir John Walton.) The 'skeletal' aspect was helped by co-operative studies with Orthopaedics (led by Prof. Paul Gregg), and the osteoporosis interests of Prof. Roger Francis.

Cawston was studying the collagenases and their inhibitors, Dr John Goodacre the possible microbial triggers of the auto-immunity in rheumatic diseases and Griffiths was leading a team concerned with Sjögren's Syndrome and other conditions. The population of Newcastle was relatively stable, favouring multi-case and family studies. Walker and his colleagues had shown that ambulatory activity was as good a measure as any of changes in bodily function in rheumatoid arthritis.

Southampton

The rheumatology service at Southampton had been built up by Dr Michael Cawley. Cawley, a 1958 St Bartholomew's graduate, was a Senior Registrar in Rheumatology at Bristol before being promoted to consultant at Wrightington hospital. He later moved back 'down South' to become Consultant to the Southampton University hospitals, a 'hands on' National Health Service appointment which he combined with appointments as Royal College of Physicians Tutor and Civilian Consultant to the Royal Naval hospital at Haslar. In 1996 he was co-author of a paper that demonstrated the superiority of nuclear magnetic resonance imaging over standard X-rays in the diagnosis of sacro-iliitis. As a general rheumatologist he had to hold the middle ground between two specialist academic units. These were: Rehabilitation, under the leadership of

Professor Lindsay McClellan, and Epidemiology, where his colleague Prof. Cyrus Cooper in the Medical Research Council Environmental Epidemiology Unit had specialised in the problems of osteoporosis, osteoarthritis and soft tissue complaints. Cooper had also studied the possible fetal programming of osteoporosis in later life.

Nottingham

At Nottingham Dr Michael Doherty who trained at Bristol was interested in pyrophosphate particles in the joint fluid in osteoarthritis and in determinants of knee pain. He is Therapeutic Professor of Rheumatology and Editor of the *Annals of Rheumatic Diseases*. His colleagues are Drs Anthony J Swannell, who trained at Bath, Hammersmith and Taplow, and Christopher Deighton who trained in Newcastle.

Leicester

Leicester was an exception in that it did not have an Arthritis and Rheumatism Council funded academic appointment. However it did have a Medical Research Council Centre for Mechanisms in Human Toxicity under Prof. Jo Lunec that was working on experimentally induced lupus and showing that agents that damage genetic DNA could be associated with development of Lupus-like antibodies to the damaged DNA.

Liverpool

The provision of services for rheumatology in Liverpool in the 1970s was disappointing to the Arthritis and Rheumatism Council (ARC) and informal negotiations were opened to see if the Medical School there could accept an ARC-endowed Professorial Chair or Lecturership. One of the Professors of Medicine, John Woodrow, an authority on genetics, ran a rheumatology outpatient clinic. He was joined in 1976 at the Royal infirmary by Dr Emlyn Williams who with fellow consultant Dr Trevor Benson set up a service in both rheumatology and rehabilitation at Fazackerly Hospital. In-patient facilities were scarce in Liverpool and yet they were much in demand because of the large pool of long neglected patients who often required prolonged periods of hospitalisation. Some had been provided for under the care of Dr Tom Littler at a converted tuberculosis hospital at Leasowe on the Wirral. It was, however, increasingly clear that Leasowe was no longer appropriate either for the long term care of ill patients or for major elective surgery. Its closure in1979 coincided with the opening of the Arrowe Park hospital on the Wirral where Dr Tom Littler established a new unit, since taken over by Dr Tom Kennedy from Charing Cross. At the Royal Liverpool Hospital Woodrow and Williams were joined in 1979 by Dr Roger Bucknall as Consultant in General Medicine who had trained in gastroenterology and after that in rheumatology at Bath and Bristol.

Discussions between the ARC, the University and Mersey Regional Hospital Authority began again in the mid-'80s. The Professors of Medicine and Surgery were supportive as was the Health Authority but the proposal for an ARC-endowed Chair of Rheumatology was not adopted. Woodrow, who was then not long off retirement, did not push for it and Bucknall felt that an academic appointment was inappropriate until better facilities were available in the Royal Liverpool Hospital for the existing clinics and their patients.

Even in the 1990 edition of the *Medical Directory* the description 'rheumatologist' was not attached to any of the staff of any of the hospitals in Liverpool. Those that did any rheumatology were listed under General Medicine and were either 'general physicians with an interest' (Woodrow and Bucknall) or undertook both rheumatology and rehabilitation (Dr Emlyn Williams). Williams suggested that this reflected the antipathy of the earlier and long influential Professor of Medicine, Lord Cohen of Birkenhead, to having 'specialists' in his department. Cohen took the view that all physicians should be able to cope with the run of general medicine but could also have a special interest. This attitude seems to have stifled the development not only of rheumatology in Liverpool but of other disciplines as well. The death of Lord Cohen in 1977 and more particularly the introduction of separate Trust status had since allowed freedom for speciality development. Williams and Dr Robert Thompson had built up the rheumatology service at Fazakerley Hospital. After Woodrow retired from the Royal Liverpool Hospital, Bucknall was joined by Dr Edward Tunn (from Professor Bacon's unit in Birmingham). Dr Tunn brought to Liverpool a much-needed computer programming expertise for keeping track of patients in Merseyside.

Fazakerley became the University Hospital at Aintree. On the campus with its large and established rheumatology service there developed a state of the art clinical facility incorporating the Walton Centre for Neurology and Neurosurgery, the Pain Relief Foundation and the University Clinical Sciences Unit. Five Professorial Chairs based on Aintree added to the first two academic appointments in rheumatology, a Lecturer and a Senior Lecturer/Honorary Consultant.

The Senior Lecturer, Dr Robert Moots, came from Birmingham via Harvard. He was the winner of the 1998 Michael Mason Prize and had been awarded an ARC grant of £120,000 to support clinical and laboratory research. His appointment had been a landmark for rheumatology in Liverpool. Elsewhere on Merseyside and in Cheshire, in an area that twenty years ago had less than three whole time equivalents in consultants in rheumatology, there were fourteen rheumatologists, one of them, Dr Joyce Davidson offering a paediatric rheumatology service. Merseyside also had six specialist rheumatology posts and was committed to providing rheumatological training to three specialist registrars in rehabilitation medicine. This was a far cry from the situation prevailing at the time of the first ARC exploratory visit in the late 1970s. There was then no system for postgraduate interchange and communication for Merseyside rheumatologists. The arrival of Malcolm Jayson as Professor of Rheumatology at Manchester saw the setting up of a Northwest Rheumatology Club that met twice a year. In addition, since 1993, there had been meetings of the Merseyside Rheumatology Club, rotating monthly between different hospitals. Attendance for trainees was mandatory. Patients were presented and problems discussed. The Trustees of ARC were keen to promote this new climate of development.

Teaching hospitals in Scotland

Aberdeen

Dr Logie Bain was born in 1914 and qualified in 1937 at Aberdeen. As a member of the Territorial Army he was called up at the outbreak of war and served until demobilised in 1945. He was appointed as Assistant Physician in Physical Medicine in Aberdeen in 1947 and invited to set up a department of Rheumatology. There were originally no beds attached to this position, only a clinic in a local swimming baths. Later beds were organised at Stracathro Hospital and he was promoted to Consultant at the Aberdeen Royal Infirmary in 1952. Bain was a prime mover in the early days of the British Arthritis Association, later called Arthritis Care, and at one time was Sheriff of Aberdeen. As other staff joined him a rheumatology group emerged that was allotted 42 beds at the City Hospital. This was reduced to 23 on moving to the Aberdeen Royal Infirmary and subsequently to 18 although the turnover of patients had doubled and the waiting time for an appointment was down to between one and six weeks. Dr Norris Rennie who trained at Aberdeen and Glasgow took over from Logie Bain when the latter retired in 1979.

Dr David Reid was Reader in Rheumatology and exemplified the development of the academic side of the Aberdeen group. He qualified in 1975 and was previously Senior Registrar at Edinburgh with Prof. George Nuki. Nuki had asked him to take charge of studies using radio-calcium and the whole body counter method in order to measure the calcium content and changes in the skeleton in rheumatic diseases. This showed that it was possible to derive the loss of bone mineral due to the disease and the additional loss in those who were treated with corticosteroids. From these early studies, Reid developed an interest in osteoporosis and was an early member of the Council of Management of the National Osteoporosis Society, later its Treasurer. Through Reid Aberdeen had a strong association with osteoporosis, notable being the work on the genetics of osteoporosis and on the methodology and effectiveness of screening and follow-up.

Reid's other colleagues in rheumatology were: Cliff Eastmond, trained at Edinburgh, Liverpool and Leeds; Alan MacDonald, trained in Glasgow and Aberdeen and Stuart Ralston, a Professor of Medicine and Therapeutics whose contact with NHS rheumatology was to do a metabolic bone disease clinic every two weeks.

Dr Norris Rennie and Dr IA Auchterlonie looked after paediatric rheumatology. For surgical rheumatology there was good co-operation and occasional joint consultative clinics with surgeons Peter Gibson and Bill Ledingham. Buchan Chesney looked after hand surgery.

Dundee

Under a scheme co-ordinated by Dr Mike Webley in Stoke Mandeville, Reid and colleagues conducted a peer review of the services for rheumatology in Dundee where Tom Pullar (ex Leeds) and Ken Morley (ex Aberdeen and Hammersmith) were consultants. Morley had taken over from Dr Mathew Wilkinson, one time trainee at Hammersmith and Charing Cross hospital, who for many years had been the sole rheumatologist for the Dundee area.

Glasgow

Early interest in the rheumatic diseases had been shown by Prof. Ralph Stockman, physician at the Western infirmary, who had published in 1920 a textbook entitled 'Rheumatism and Arthritis'. It was the same Stockman who believed that the condition called fibrositis or fibromyalgia was an expression of inflammation of the

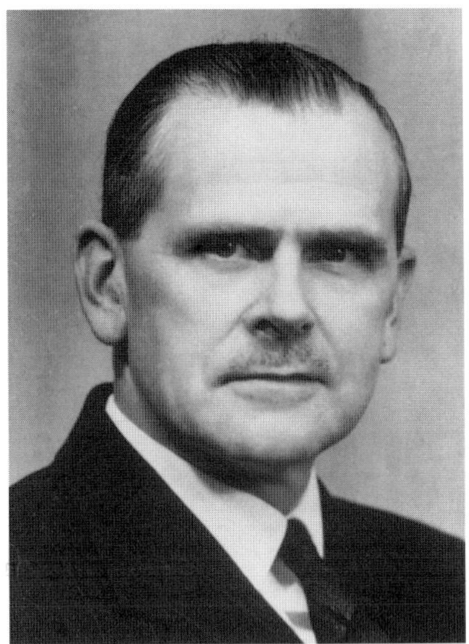
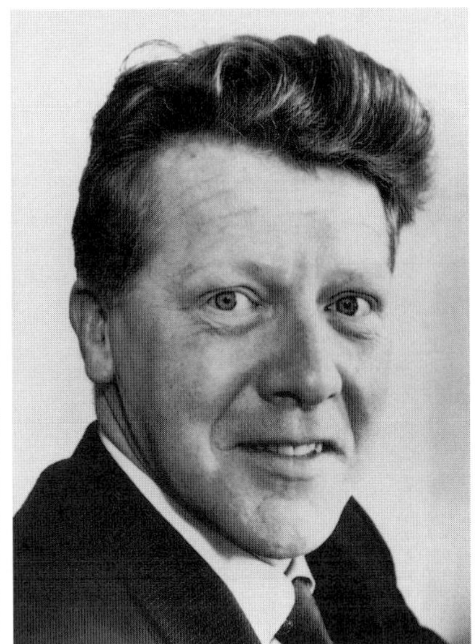

Fig 4.1. Left, Dr Tom Fraser. Right, Dr JP Currie

fibrous tissue in muscles. Others have concluded that he extrapolated from a patient who had dermatomyositis. Another physician interested in rheumatic conditions was Dr James Reid whose son became Regius Professor of Medicine at Glasgow University. Reid senior wrote a series of articles on salicylates and related compounds in relation to rheumatic fever.

There was no establishment of consultant posts in Physical Medicine in Glasgow at the end of the war when Dr Tom Fraser and Dr J P Currie (Figs 4.1) looked after rheumatology. Fraser had graduated from Glasgow in 1933 and was a pioneer in the treatment of rheumatoid arthritis with gold therapy. He had a rheumatism unit at the Killearn Hospital and was a full physician at the Western Infirmary. Currie (*Lancet,* 1952), was the first in the UK to describe treatment with phenylbutazone. (He also used it in a veterinary capacity, treating the horse 'Merely-a-Monarch', a show jumper owned by A Drummond Hay. Known as 'Bute', it was to become a favourite veterinary medicine).

In the late 1950s Tom Fraser was not a well man and Currie did not have the academic credentials acceptable to the university authorities. It was decided to set up a specialist rheumatology department.

Glasgow was the one city in the UK where modern academic rheumatology was *not* started by one of the trainees of the first three professors. Dr William Watson Buchanan had trained at Glasgow and qualified in 1954. He started to specialise in endocrinology but was impressed with the concept of auto-immune disease after investigating a patient who had both rheumatoid arthritis and autoimmune thyroiditis. He went to Bethesda on a scholarship and worked with Dr JJ Bunim on the Sjögren's or 'sicca' syndrome, also on intradermal injection of micro-crystalline sodium urate in an attempt to elucidate some of the features of gout. Returning to Glasgow in

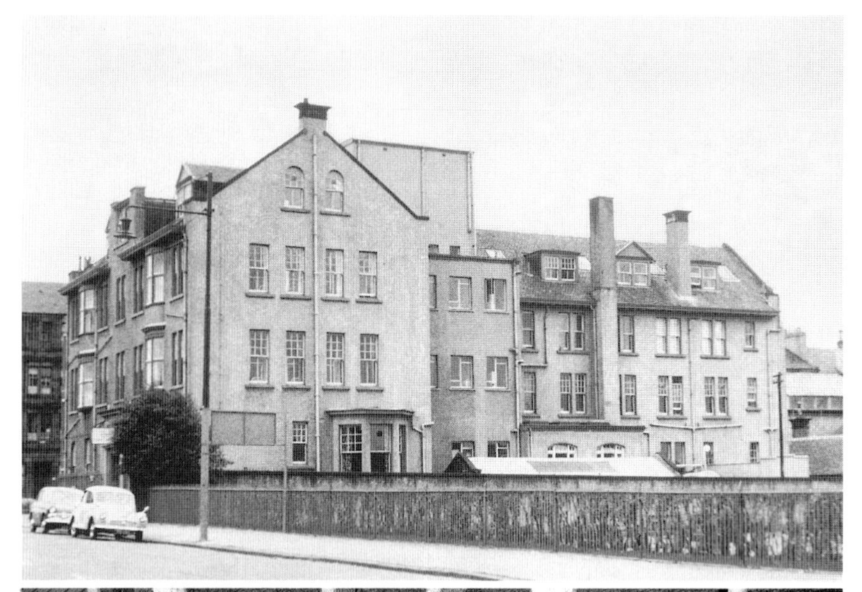

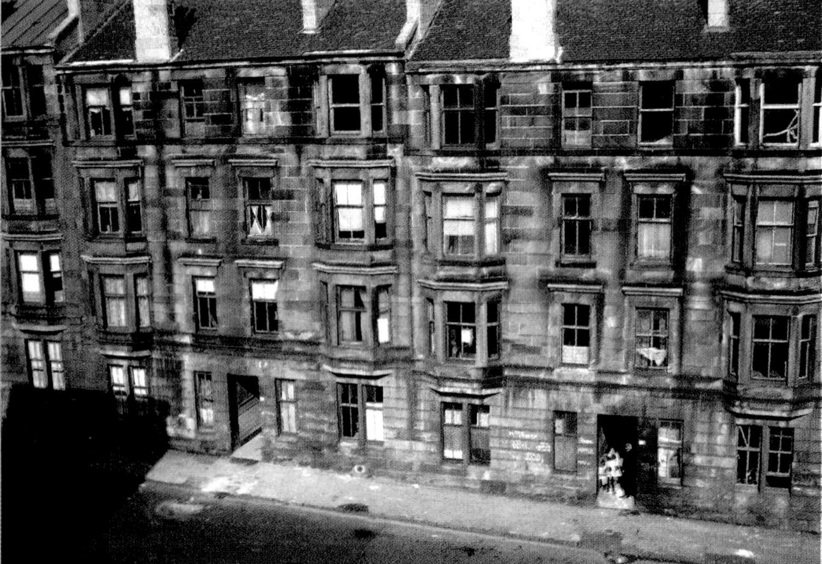

Fig 4.2. The Centre for Rheumatic Diseases in Baird Street, Glasgow, opposite slum tenements.

1964 he was appointed Consultant in the Rheumatic Diseases at an ex-tuberculosis hospital in Baird Street in Glasgow, (Fig 4.2) opposite slum tenements and he built it up into an internationally famous centre despite some indifference from his University colleagues. He attracted bright young trainees, many of them from abroad and paid for by their governments. He sent his UK trainees to Egypt, Eastern Europe and Portugal to make bridges with rheumatology there. With Dr Tony Boyle he produced a textbook of Rheumatology which was well received. In 1972 he was made Professor. In 1976 he organised a meetting of the Heberden Society and gave the Heberden Round.

He was vociferous in his opposition to any compromise between rheumatology and physical medicine. Figure 4.3 is a copy of a slide of the hierarchy of Medicine throwing rheumatology to the sharks that he showed at the meeting.

So how was it that one year later his University colleagues were so antagonised that his backers Sir Edward Wayne and Sir Charles Illingworth, by then retired but still influential, advised him that he should resign and move to Canada?

Perhaps some indication can be got from the enormous research output (over 250 scientific papers and contributions to books) and the numbers of trainees (19), who passed through the Centre between1964 and 1977. It gives the impression of a young man in a hurry and on his own admission Buchanan could spare little time for bureaucrats and committees. This was to be his Achilles heel. 'Not going through official channels' started soon after he was appointed when he ordered the architect to arrange for an immunology laboratory to be built but had not first obtained official authorisation. It continued when he appointed a second and unauthorised Registrar in the early days. He could not get the authorities of the Health Board to provide an out-patient department and in-house Xray facilities despite vocal protests which did not endear him to them. He protected himself by forming an Arthritis Society Committee which included leaders of local industry, the Catholic Archbishop (who had gout), the Protestant Professor of Theology, and the Chairman of the Rangers Football Club.

In 1977 it was World Rheumatism Year. Officials of the Greater Glasgow Health Board celebrated it in Glasgow by the attempted closure of the Centre for Rheumatic Diseases. Buchanan had had a written notice that that this was to be

Fig 4.3. Rheumatalogy and Physical Medicine: Watson Buchanan's concept.

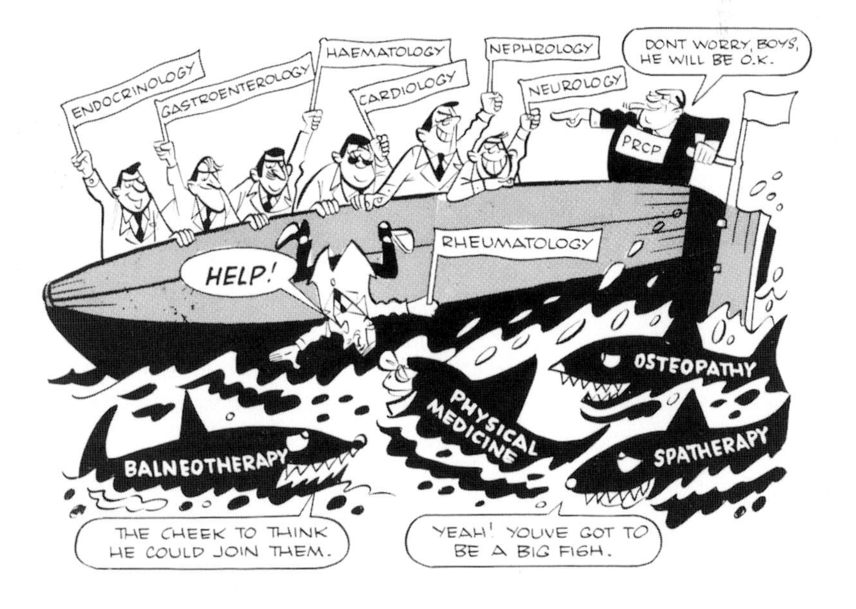

discussed but he had not read it until the meeting was already in progress. He hurried to the meeting but when he got there it was too late; the decision had already been taken. When asked by a nurse in the Centre how things had gone, he told her. The patients heard about it and 'Then all hell broke out' They wrote 200 letters to the Glasgow Herald and when they were not published they phoned the Herald office blocking all lines. The Editor gave in, published six letters and wrote a scathing editorial criticising the Board.

One patient wrote to the Prime Minister, had questions asked in the House of Commons, appeared nightly on Scottish Television and appealed to the European Court of Human Rights. Other patients wrote to the Duke of Edinburgh who phoned the Secretary of State for Scotland and indicated that he would intervene if the closure went through.

The authorities had to give in. He got his Out-patients and X-rays. Buchanan emphasised that he had not initiated nor supported the revolt as was erroneously reported and widely believed, but then neither had he attempted to stop it. So he got the blame. Administrative animus was such that things became increasingly difficult. He realised it would be better to leave. A job in Hamilton, Ontario, beckoned. He discussed it with Sir Edward Wayne and Sir Charles Illingworth and they advised him to take it. In 1978 he resigned and built up an internationally famous rheumatology service in McMaster University..

Shortly after he left, the University received £500,000 for rheumatology research, the McFarlane Bequest.

After Buchanan left Dr.Carson Dick was temporarily in charge but transferred to Newcastle in January 1979. There was a gap until 1st June 1979 when Dr Roger Sturrock, Senior Lecturer in Rheumatology at the Westminster Medical School was appointed. He was one of those who had shared in the 1972 Robecchi prize for rheumatology awarded by the European League against Rheumatism. His first action was to promote Dr Hilary Capell to Consultant for her to analyse the long-term effects of disease modifying drugs in rheumatoid arthritis.

The hospital in Baird Street closed in 1984 when the Centre for Rheumatic Diseases moved to the Glasgow Royal Infirmary. In 1990 a combination of the McLeod bequest and Arthritis and Rheumatism Council funding endowed a Chair at Glasgow with Sturrock the current holder.

Three hospital trusts had evolved in Glasgow from mergers: Acute, North of the Clyde; Acute, South of the Clyde and a separate trust for the Hospital for Sick Children (RHSC) where Dr Krishna Goel was interested in paediatric rheumatology and with whom Sturrock did a monthly clinic. This was helpful with unusual conditions such as Kawasaki's Disease and chronic pain syndromes in children. There were negotiations to set up a tertiary referral centre for paediatric rheumatology for the whole of Scotland based at the RHSC.

Prof. Eddie Liew at the Western Infirmary provided immunology support for research into cytokines IL-15 and IL-18 and their role in inflammation. Other co-operative studies concerned joint proprioception and newer methods of imaging joints and muscles.

Glasgow traditionally 'looked after' rheumatology for the immediate population centre and for Western Scotland. Rehabilitation was represented by facilities for young chronic sick and head injuries at the Department of Medical Rehabilitation at the Southern Hospital.

All but three of the district general hospitals that looked to Glasgow for expertise were by 1998 provided with at least one rheumatologist. Whereas in Edinburgh there was only one academic unit in the catchment area, the 'Hub and Spokes' principle in Glasgow, because of the two hospital trusts, had two 'hubs', the Western and the Royal Infirmaries. There were plans to make undergraduate experience in rheumatology part of general medicine. Previously there had been a 'block' system with a lecture in the fourth year

Sturrock continued the policy started by Buchanan of fostering contacts abroad. Links have been reopened with Hungary (Budapest, Prof. Geza Balint) and new ones forged with the Ukraine.

Teaching hospital in Wales

Cardiff

The National Health Service was born in the valleys of South Wales. Aneurin Bevan before he became Minister of Health in 1946 had been associated with the Tredegar Workman's Medical Aid Fund and had served on the Tredegar Hospital Management Committee. In Parliament he represented Ebbw Vale in the post war Labour government. He was well aware of the longing of the ordinary people for protection against disease and also of the fierce loyalty in the Welsh mining valleys to their local hospitals. Those hospitals had been built and supported by the efforts and the 'penny in the pound' contributions of the miners and steelworkers even during the hardest times of unemployment and strikes. Nevertheless Bevan took a larger view. One of his first tasks was to introduce the National Health Service Bill that became the 1946 Act. By ministerial order he established thirteen Hospital Regions in England, but only one for Wales and Monmouthshire. There would be at least one teaching hospital to each region, and district general hospitals would look to the teaching hospitals for clinical expertise and postgraduate leadership. Small hospitals such as those in the Welsh valleys would inevitably be downgraded in importance as a result. There was of course opposition. Bevan understood that but in Parliament said:

"...There is a tendency in some quarters to defend the very small hospital on the grounds of its localism and intimacy, and for other rather imponderable reasons of that sort, but everybody knows today that if a hospital is to be efficient it most provide a number of specialised services".

"Although I am not myself a devotee of bigness for bigness sake, I would rather be kept alive in the efficient if cold altruism of a large hospital than expire in a gush of warm sympathy in a small one."
(Hansard, 30 April 1946)

The designation of the whole of Wales and Monmouthshire as one hospital region may have reflected Welsh nationalism but it did not match previous patterns of hospital referral. The inhabitants of North Wales looked to Oswestry,

Chester, Liverpool or Manchester for specialist advice because of limited road and rail communications with Cardiff. In South East Wales and Monmouth, the Severn tunnel made it relatively easy to get to Bristol or Bath: even more so when the first Severn bridge was opened in 1966.

Before the war, as in the rest of the United Kingdom, treatment for chronic rheumatic diseases in Wales was physical treatment that took place in the two surviving Welsh Spas, Builth Wells and Llandrindod Wells, or in the physical medicine departments of the main hospitals. In Cardiff patients would be referred to the Department of Physical Medicine. This, after the National Health Service Act became law in 1948, was under the direction of Dr Kenneth Lloyd.

Lloyd trained at the London Hospital and qualified in 1938. When war came he joined the Royal Air Force Volunteer Reserve as Squadron Leader Medical Specialist and looked after the fighter pilots during the Battle of Britain in 1940. Later postings took him to the Middle East and the Royal Air Force Hospital in Cairo. He was demobilised in 1946 and returned to the London Hospital Department of Physical Medicine to work with Dr Will Tegner. He also held a weekly clinic at the West London Hospital with Dr WSC Copeman.

In 1948 when he was appointed to the Cardiff Royal Infirmary and the Llandough Hospital his title was Physician-in-charge of the Physical Medicine Department. As such he promoted the idea that the schools of Physiotherapy, Occupational Therapy and Nursing should share one building and by implication share a common introductory course of studies. The heads of these schools would not have it, although they were persuaded to share a new building. At first Lloyd had no 'teaching' beds for admitting patients and this meant that bedside teaching of medical students about rheumatic diseases was undertaken by physicians or medical registrars with an interest in rheumatology, including Drs Idris Jones and Dr Brian McConkey, who later moved to Birmingham. But things were to change as Lloyd increasingly identified himself more with rheumatology than physical medicine.

Fig 4.4. Dr Kenneth Lloyd in 1998

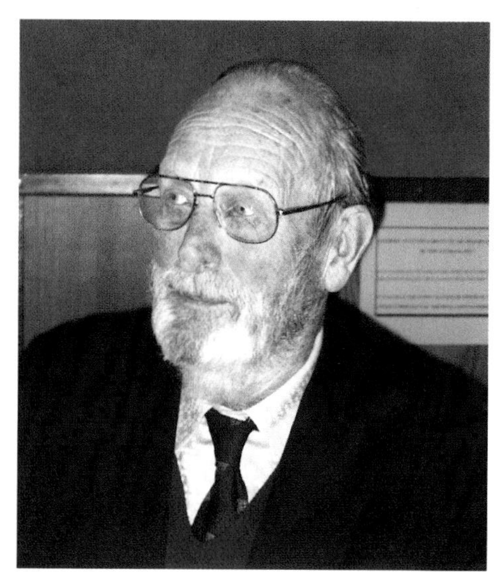

Lloyd became the first Chairman of a fund raising committee of the Arthritis and Rheumatism Council that was established in Cardiff following a visit by Dr. Will Copeman in 1960. Lloyd's wife, Phyllis, was appointed Chairman of the Ladies Committee. Sir Kenneth Treharne, Lord Lieutenant of Glamorgan, was the first President. The committees worked hard, assisted by group secretaries and organisers and the number of support committees increased throughout Wales. The change of emphasis from physical medicine to rheumatology was marked by the appointment of Dr John Jessop as second consultant rheumatologist in Cardiff in 1971 (second also in the whole of Wales). When the University Hospital of Wales at the Heath Park site was opened in 1972 and the Infirmary closed, Lloyd's title was changed to Consultant Rheumatologist. Lloyd (fig 4.4), assisted by Jessop together with the orthopaedic surgeons designed a combined orthopaedic and rheumatology out-patient suite for the new teaching hospital, with adjacent teaching rooms permitting easy interchanging of patients and ideas, leading to regular combined clinics. An 8-bedded rheumatology ward, offices and facilities for physiotherapy, occupational therapy and hydrotherapy were provided. There were also 23 beds at the Llandough Hospital in west Cardiff. Cardiff was thus able to act as a referral centre for the whole of South Wales.

As a University hospital it needed an academic presence. With the support of the Arthritis and Rheumatism Council a small rheumatology laboratory was built at Llandough Hospital when Dr George Nuki was appointed in 1974 as Senior Lecturer. In 1979 Lloyd retired and was succeeded by Dr Michael Pritchard and in the same year Nuki resigned to become ARC Professor of Rheumatology in Edinburgh. The Llandough rheumatology laboratories were expanded with the aid of a further grant from the Arthritis and Rheumatism Council. In 1982 Dr Bryan Williams was appointed Senior Lecturer in Rheumatology within the Department of Medicine with academic facilities on the University Hospital of Wales site at Heath Park.

The combination of additional staff and facilities and the integration of rheumatology services within the University Hospital and Llandough Hospital had the benefits of immediate expert advice from colleagues in other disciplines, facilities for sharing and rotating junior staff between departments and opportunities for multidisciplinary research projects. The attraction of trainee doctors to the field of rheumatology increased and between 1971 and 1998 the number of consultant rheumatologists in Wales increased from two to seventeen.

The rheumatology department under the direction of Lloyd and later Jessop initiated a number of high quality research studies. An early study was on the effect of iron dextran in rheumatoid arthritis. The authors observed that the material could temporarily increase pain, an important observation to be attributed 20 years later to the release by the iron of active oxygen radicals in areas of inflammation. Jessop in retirement continued his work on the fifth year of follow-up of a randomised trial of four different second-line drugs used for the treatment of rheumatoid arthritis, hydroxychloroquine, sodium aurothiomallate, auranofin, and penicillamine The study achieved a uniquely high completion rate with few drop-outs after five years. Penicillamine emerged as the most practical long-term treatment.

After 1972 services linked to rheumatology could improve. Back pain problems, as elsewhere in the United Kingdom at the time, had been 'orphan' complaints that were referred to consultants in various different specialities. There was no service dedicated solely to back pain. Jessop described the services for rehabilitation of rheumatic disease patients in 1971 as less than satisfactory. Llandaff Rookwood Hospital had up to the 1970s been an Armed Services rehabilitation hospital. It included a spinal injuries unit. It had in the past taken in rheumatology in-patients for rehabilitation but not on a regular basis. Since then rehabilitation has improved with the work of Dr K T Rajan at Pontypridd. Dr George Nuki and paediatrician Dr Tal Thomas built up a paediatric rheumatology service and Dr Molly Hall and paediatrician Dr Corrie Weaver expanded this at Rookwood and Caerphilly hospitals, later at Cardiff. As a result the University Hospital of Wales at Cardiff became recognised as a centre of excellence within this sub-speciality. Hall retired in 1997. Her general rheumatology work had been taken over by Dr Sharon Jones, previously at Bath, and her paediatric rheumatology by Dr J Camilleri. Lupus immunology and the connective tissue diseases that had been the concern of Dr George Nuki before he moved to Edinburgh had been taken over by Bryan Williams, who became Reader and was appointed to the first Chair of Rheumatology in Wales in 1995.

The first combined orthopaedic/rheumatology clinics were held in 1972 with Mr Michael Young, newly appointed consultant orthopaedic surgeon. Over the years technical advances had led to improvements in the procedures available. There was a huge demand and combined clinics were held monthly. When Young retired the service was split into upper and lower limb surgery. Nuki and plastic surgeon Mr Philip Sykes took over the hand surgery. Mr Chris Wilson gave 'superb service' (Jessop) for lower limb surgery.

By the 1990s there was good co-operation in the 'general medical' aspects of rheumatology with cardiac, ophthalmic and dermatologist colleagues through normal intra-hospital consultation. An ankylosing spondylitis clinic had been set up. It aimed to see patients at least once a year.

Cardiff became famous for its record in epidemiology under the late Dr Archie Cochrane. John Lawrence had worked with him in his studies of rheumatic complaints in the Rhondda Fach. Arising out of the epidemiological interest in coal miners' pneumoconiosis, Dr A Caplan had noted in 1953 that the lung disease presented atypically as rounded shadows on chest X-ray in miners who also had, *or were later to develop,* rheumatoid arthritis. This was important and compelling evidence that rheumatoid arthritis could 'throw a shadow before' and there might therefore be a rheumatoid diathesis.

The staff contributed to the national and local support organisations in rheumatology. Jessop served on the committees of Arthritis Care (AC), the British League against Rheumatism and the Arthritis and Rheumatism Council (ARC). Dr Michael Pritchard looked after the local support group of the ARC. In Cardiff, unlike in some other centres, the local support organisations of the ARC and AC were separate.

Since 1971 it had been the policy of the Specialist Advisory Sub-Committee in Rheumatology to persuade the Welsh Medical Committee and Manpower Committee of the need for more consultant posts in rheumatology. These would be based in each District Hospital in Wales. In 1992 the Welsh Medical Committee set up a Working Party to advise on 'Recommendations for Service provision and Good practice for People with Rheumatism and Arthritis in Wales'. The Welsh Medical Committee and the Chief Medical Officer for Wales accepted the Working Party's recommendations in 1995. Despite this there were no consultant rheumatology posts in

West Wales, especially Dyfed, and inadequate provision in North and West Wales (Jessop). Nevertheless, rheumatologists had been appointed to all the bigger hospitals in Wales and the 'hub and spokes' principle was taking effect in most of them.

Committees in Cardiff may recommend but after the 'provider-purchaser' reforms power to make changes at hospital level resided with the local Trusts and their administrators. The Cardiff rheumatologists had themselves experienced this. They had seen a gross reduction in beds available to them and the dismantling of their out-patient department at the University Hospital of Wales to make way for an endoscopy Unit.

Rheumatology had made little progress in Gwent. The target provision for Wales had been one rheumatologist for every 100,000 persons. Glamorgan had nearly reached this with three whole time equivalents for a population of 400,000. For Gwent the ratio was only 1 to 400,000. As a result, Gwent had to rely on 'bought out' services from neighbouring trusts.

In order to rationalise the situation Gwent, after the introduction of the purchaser/provider relationship, put its rheumatological services out to tender. The tender was won by a combined bid from Nevill Hall Hospital in Abergavenny and the Royal National Hospital for Rheumatic Diseases in Bath in a contract which extended until March 2000. Two new consultants, Drs Tim Jenkinson and Andrew Borg were appointed.

Understandably the authorities in Cardiff were somewhat put out by this development in what was traditionally 'their' territory and at first the newcomers were given a reserved reception. Arrangements had been made to merge Nevill Hall, Abergavenny and the Royal Gwent hospitals into one trust when the five-year contract with Bath ended. Jessop hoped that this would lead to an improvement, not just in rheumatology service but in academic rheumatology as well.

There was a long history of exchange between Bath and Wales. In 1970 one quarter of all in-patients at the Royal National Hospital for Rheumatic Diseases came from South Wales. In 1995 colleagues in Bangor, North Wales, invited Prof Peter Maddison from Bath to consider moving to Bangor to help develop rheumatology services there and he accepted. He was learning Welsh 'so that I can hear what people are saying about me when they think I don't understand!'

There were worries that this development might loosen the already tenuous links between North Wales and Cardiff. North and South Wales had some cultural differences, particularly in the proportion of the population that was Welsh speaking. Transport and communication difficulties in the past had meant that it was easier for a rheumatism sufferer from Northeast Wales to be referred to Oswestry, the Wirral, Liverpool or even London (less than 4 hours by through train from Bangor to Euston) than to Cardiff (by train at least two changes and taking five hours)

Moreover, the academic structure in Wales was unusual. All separate colleges throughout Wales came under the overall heading of the University of Wales in which Cardiff had the dominant position and could attract the best A-level students, to the point where some academics in Cardiff had urged that these other colleges be 'de-merged'. However at a professional level, rheumatologists in Wales had a strong and cohesive association that met twice a year, alternating between north and south. Additionally, 'cross border' professional exchanges took place in the regular meetings of the West Country, Wessex and South Wales Rheumatology Club and at the conferences of the British Society for Rheumatology. At the political level, it remained to be seen how Aneurin Bevan's heritage of a single Welsh Hospital Region with centralised control would react to the transfer of power to individual hospital trusts and their managers.

Teaching hospital in Northern Ireland.

Belfast

Northern Ireland in 1948 had a population of about $1^1/_2$ million concentrated in Belfast and environs and a handful of other cities. In the countryside and coasts there were many small hospitals with less than 100 beds. Tourism as an industry had not started then and was later discouraged by the 'troubles'.

The setting in which rheumatology developed in Northern Ireland was much the same as in mainland Britain. In Belfast the Royal Victoria Hospital was the voluntary teaching hospital but the Belfast City Hospital was the workhouse type of establishment.

In the 1940s Sir Thomas Houston at the Royal Victoria Hospital prepared autologous vaccines from the nasopharyngeal swabs of patients with rheumatoid arthritis and these were administered by Dr Campbell Young, a general practitioner, in the waiting area of the old out-patient department. A Dr Duffield and a surgeon Colonel Dan McVicar practised manipulative therapy on the Cyriax model, but general physicians or orthopaedic surgeons saw the bulk of rheumatic disease patients.

Dr William Lennon was Physician to Outpatients in the Royal Victoria Hospital before the war. After war service he trained with Dr CB Heald at the Royal Free Hospital. When he returned to Belfast he found his efforts to set up a service for rheumatism patients were resisted by his medical colleagues. He was relegated to a small room in the basement of the hospital. His beds were in a convalescent hospital some three miles away. He practised conventional rheumatology using gold injections together with oral and intra-articular corticosteroids. He was never made a Fellow of the Royal College. "Which says something of his colleagues at the Infirmary!" - Dr Walter Boyd.

The first of today's rheumatologists was Boyd who qualified in 1943 and after war service did a post release year at the Belfast City hospital where a number of patients with advanced rheumatoid disease stimulated his interest in the field. He undertook postgraduate training with Bywaters at Hammersmith and Taplow and visits to Kellgren and Duthie.

After junior appointments Boyd became Registrar Tutor to Professor Graham Bull in the Department of Medicine in the Royal Victoria Hospital. He was promoted to Consultant General Physician at Belfast City and Musgrave Park hospitals with a declared interest in establishing a rheumatic disease service alongside the existing orthopaedic service. Musgrave Park had before the war been a reform school for wayward boys who were trained as naval cadets. During the war it was taken over as an Emergency Medical Services hospital. Rheumatology was allotted a Nissen hut type ward that had previously housed tuberculosis patients.

When Dr Lennon retired Dr Stanley Roberts replaced him. Roberts had also been to Hammersmith and Taplow for postgraduate training in rheumatology.

To accommodate this at the Musgrave Park Hospital, a further half Nissen Hut was added to give a total of 60 beds. Together Boyd and Roberts founded the Irish Society for Rheumatology[7]. From 1960 onwards the Belfast rheumatologists provided a regional service for the whole of Northern Ireland. By 1990 there were five rheumatologists, all in the Eastern Region of the Health and Social Services Board. Since then the numbers had risen to nine, as services became available in the other regions of the province and specialist clinics were opened up. Dr Aubrey Bell looked after paediatric rheumatology and there were good services for surgical rheumatology.

Boyd's publication list reflected his transition from general medicine to rheumatology. Until 1977 it included papers on endocrine topics. After that there were papers on aspects of rheumatic diseases and their treatment. An early paper that exemplified the change illustrated the rheumatoid-like hand deformities of Werner's syndrome of precocious aging, a rare condition that might present with diabetes and hypogonadism (Boyd, 1959).

Dr Stanley Roberts gave the Heberden Round in 1995 and Roberts was later elected President of the Royal College of Physicians of Ireland, a striking contrast to the treatment of Dr Lennon 50 years earlier.

A visitor to Northern Ireland in 2000 would find it looking prosperous with new buildings everywhere, a prosperity underpinned with money from the European Union. Where else in the United Kingdom than Belfast would one find a major city that was approached by a ten lane highway? Unmanned police road-blocks on the borders with Eire are the only visible reminders of past religious and political tensions.

7 It was originally to be called the Irish Rheumatism Association but the initials were considered infelicitous.

Chapter 5.
Rheumatology and the Spa Hospitals.

The history of the spas of Europe is the history of Europe itself. One can speculate that mankind, like sparrows, has an instinct for communal immersion and splashing about, whether it be for religious reasons in the Ganges or for social reasons in the great Diocletian baths of 3rd century Rome. Wherever in Europe the Roman soldiers came, they constructed baths for the conquerors and the rehabilitation of their legions. From Aqua Gratianae (Aix-les-Bains) to Aqua Sulis (Bath) hundreds of spas were established.

When the Romans left, many spas survived and as the population and wealth of Europe grew so did the number of spas. The waters in the spas were believed to have great healing virtues and medicinal properties. One could swallow it, be sprayed with it, bath in it singly or communally, or have it administered as a clyster or colonic irrigation. Spa waters were -still are- bottled or barreled and transported for sale and use elsewhere. Some spa waters did have medicinal properties. Epsom is remembered today for its laxative Epsom Salts, (magnesium sulphate). Sulphur-containing waters helped certain skin diseases.

Most spa sources are based on fossil water. That which arises in Bath and in Hotwells in Bristol probably fell on the hills of Northern Ireland thousands of years ago. It trickles down to a source of heat in the earth's mantle and loses specific gravity as it heats up and finds its way to an egress at a lower elevation. The source of heat is either vulcanic as in Rotorua or radioactive as in Bath. The mineral content of the water depends on the subterranean beds through which the water passes on its way to the surface. Where there had been ancient volcanic activity the water might be sulphurous, as at Strathpeffer. Coming through an ancient dried up lagoon it would contain brine, as at Droitwich. Whatever their chemical nature, spa waters shared the property of buoyancy which helped stiff and crippled limbs to move and was the reason why spa therapy before 1948 was almost synonymous with the treatment of rheumatism.

The magic of water gushing out of the ground inspired religious wells and religious faith in their powers of healing. Faith is a major component of motivation. In turn, motivationis an apt word for the will to keep joints moving despite pain.

The height of the popularity of the spas was in the eighteenth and nineteenth centuries. The rich flocked to them and built or rented their summer holiday homes by them. Londoners would go to Bath or Tunbridge Wells much as today's Londoners would rent or buy a property in the Algarve. The spas developed pleasure gardens, assembly rooms and places to eat where the rich and elegant could parade or meet. To divert them there were theatres, gaming houses and racecourses. To see to their souls there were churches. To look after the sick who sought relief from their illnesses there were hospitals and medical men.

At one time there were at least ten spas and watering places in London with others such as Tunbridge Wells easily reachable in a day's journey by coach and horses and later by railway. Alderson (1973) lists over 80 spas and 'spa-lets' in Britain.

Of these only a few remain. Sadler's Wells are remembered because of the theatre, Battersea Gardens for their pleasure grounds, Epsom for its Derby. Royal Leamington Spa and Woodhall Spa are now only place names. In Bath, Buxton, Droitwich and Harrogate the hospitals associated with the spas were taken over by the Health Service in 1948 but the civic Spa facilities remained outside it.

In Europe the civic spas together with their hospitals came under the direction of the national tourists agencies. In Europe the civic spas prospered. In the UK they for practical purposes disappeared. In his book 'Spas That Heal', the late WAR Thompson, one time Editor of *The Practitioner*, raged against the burghers and doctors in the Spa towns who let the spas dwindle and disappear [Thompson, 1978]. In truth there was little the doctors could have done other than in their private capacity as citizens.

Droitwich, The Highfield and St John's Hospitals

Droitwich is a town situated over large rock salt deposits that have been exploited since before Roman times. In 1836, after the discovery of a subterranean brine stream, entrepreneurs opened the Royal Brine Baths, later (1887) the St Andrew's Brine Baths provided hydrotherapy treatments until 1971 when the local council bought the building and closed it down. The patients were transferred to the Highfield Hospital that with its associated St John's Hospital provided 120 beds for rheumatic disease patients, most of them from Birmingham. Highfield was linked to rheumatology in the University of Birmingham Queen Elizabeth Hospital with Professor Paul Bacon as visiting Consultant. The expanding town of Droitwich had planned to replace its historic Spa with a health and sports complex but this never came to fruition. The heated brine swimming pool, which had survived the closure of the St Andrew's Baths, itself closed in 1976.

For patients with rheumatoid arthritis and for others with weak or painful limbs, the major benefit of heated brine over ordinary water was the increase in buoyancy, making it even easier to move and re-train damaged muscles and joints. A disadvantage was the need for a subsequent fresh water shower to remove residual salt. A possible danger was the accidental inhalation of a drop of brine, which could set up laryngeal spasm.

Medical supervision of the Spa facilities at Droitwich was originally under the care of Dr 'Pat' Patterson, who, like Dr Kersley of Bath, would travel regularly to Peto Place in London to see patients and arrange for their treatment in the Spa. He was joined in 1964 by Dr John Popert, who had trained in rheumatology at the West London Hospital and later at the Manchester Royal Infirmary with Professor Kellgren. He is the author of a study widely cited at the time on the epidemiology of gout and hyperuricaemia and he subsequently championed the use of hydroxychloroquin and chloroquine for rheumatoid arthritis. He was also an early advocate of the use of cytotoxic drugs for the more severe expressions of rheumatoid arthritis. He has tried a variety of these agents. Best, in his experience, was nitrogen mustard.

Dr Popert did his best to save the historic Spa facility but it was felt (in Birmingham) that the citizens of Birmingham would be better provided for if the

Droitwich services were moved to Redditch. The advent of Trust status for hospitals frustrated this when the Worcester group of hospitals gained independence from Birmingham. Instead, rheumatology was transferred to a 12-bedded unit in the Worcester Royal Infirmary under the care of Dr Ian Rowe and the Highfields and St John's hospitals closed in 1994.

Asked how he viewed the destruction of the hospitals where he had worked, Popert said that it was a disaster for the patients. Rheumatoid arthritis patients needed and deserved something more than a quick fix 'bolus' cocktail of methotrexate and methylprednisolone administered as an out-patient or after a minimal period of admission. Much effort had gone into the Droitwich hospitals to improve the service. Much money had been raised to support these improvements and he deplored the expunging of all he had worked for. He suspected that those who should have supported the Highfield and St John's Hospitals had had a hidden agenda that involved developing Redditch at the expense of Droitwich.

A brine bath facility and hydrotherapy unit was reopened in Droitwich in 1986. It became incorporated in a private hospital. The public can use this, but have to pay.

Harrogate, the Royal Bath Hospital.

'Harrogate has sold its heritage for a mess of potage' (Thompson, 1978). Thompson goes on to trace the history of the different springs and sources, sulphurous, chalybeate or alum containing and the rising popularity of the city as a spa town as these were increasingly exploited. 'On an August day in 1911 there were no less than three queens in the Spa, Queen Alexandra, Empress Marie of Russia, and the Queen of Portugal'. A hospice for the sick poor was built in 1826. It was replaced by the grand new Royal Baths Hospital in Cornwall Road in1887. The Royal Baths in the centre of the town were opened in 1897 and closed in 1969.

The Royal Bath Hospital was an important military rehabilitation centre during the Second World War. In 1924 funds had been raised to build a research centre in the hospital grounds. When visited in 1960, there were then the historic Royal Bath Hospital with 130 beds, the Rawson Miners' Convalescent Home next door and the White Hart Hospital, a converted hotel near the Spa centre, altogether about 300 beds for rheumatology and rehabilitation. The position of consultant rheumatologist was on offer at the time. Plus values about the job were: the support of the local community; access to the research laboratory where pathologist Douglas Collins had worked; the large number of patients ensuring a wide clinical experience and the link with the Leeds General Infirmary. The connection with Leeds University was through Professor Stanley Hartfall, joked about at the time as the 'only man in Yorkshire known to be able to turn gold into brass', a reflection of his championing the use of gold treatment of rheumatoid arthritis in his private patients. Prof Ronald Tunbridge of the Leeds Medical School was clearly at odds with Hartfall. Tunbridge said that because of the attitude and non-co-operation of Hartfall, Leeds had lost the support of the Oliver Bird money that it might have expected.

Dr Yeoman, Physician to the Royal Bath Hospital, recalled an interesting adverse effect of going to a spa for treatment. The youngest example of gout he had seen was in a girl of twelve whose parents had met when they had accompanied their parents to the Harrogate Spa. Both the grandfathers were seeking treatment for familial gout. An instance of unnatural selection?

Dr Howard Bird was appointed as Consultant to the Leeds General Infirmary in 1980 assisting Professor Verna Wright. His duties included looking after in-patients in the Royal Bath Hospital at Harrogate. He took over the laboratory block whence Douglas Collins had published the first book on the pathology of the rheumatic diseases. There Bird set up the Rheumatology Clinical Pharmacology Unit with backing from the Swiss firm of Roche. As part of this he saw the need for the training and qualification of the specialist nurses and physiotherapists (called Clinical Metrologists) who were responsible for filling in the primary data on the clinical trial forms for the study of new antirheumatic drugs. He also pointed to the possible fallacies of the system of self assessment in which a patient was asked to place a mark on a line between 0 and 100 to indicate her perception of pain or pain relief. There was an innate tendency to point to the 'Golden Section.'

Howard Bird predicted that the future for drug evaluation would call for large-scale clinical trials conducted by numerous co-operating centres so to enhance statistical power. Regulatory authorities were insisting on immaculate quality control of primary data. Form filling would take away some of the enthusiasm for this work compared with the days when one centre could be wholly responsible for a published study.

In 1974 the White Hart Hospital closed, ostensibly on the grounds that it was unsafe, only to be shortly re-opened as a conference hotel for the administrators. Beds in the Royal Bath Hospital were gradually reduced so that by 1990 there were 97 beds [*Medical Directory figures*] falling to 57 at the time of closure of the hospital. This did not reflect deliberate policy so much as a reaction to the growth of rheumatological services elsewhere in the Yorkshire region. Thus Maurice Jefferies lost his beds in the Royal Bath Hospital when the Bradford authorities decided they could manage more cheaply without them. Michael Martin, Consultant at St. James Teaching Hospital in Leeds, arranged to withdraw his sessions in 1987, one reason being the absence of orthopaedic surgery at Harrogate, together with the falling number of referrals. The truth was that the hospital was dying long before it finally closed. Only Prof. Wright's unit remained faithful to the end. His psoriatic arthritis register was based there, together with some of the bioengineering work with Bahaa Seedhom. When the Leeds Hospital Trust withdrew Leeds-funded patients from Harrogate it sealed the fate of the Royal Bath Hospital. It closed in 1994 and in 1998 was partly demolished and surrounded by scaffolding. Flats were being built behind the original façade. The proceeds would help fund Harrogate's hospital and medical services. There was some opposition to this from local preservation societies but not strong enough to save the hospital. The physicians who worked there have dispersed, Wendy Dodds to Lancaster, Howard Bird to a purpose built unit in Chapel Allerton Hospital where he has a Chair in Developmental Pharmacological Rheumatology, Michael Martin to St James Hospital in Leeds, and Martin Iveson to York. There does not seem to have been the sense of loss that accompanied the closing of the Droitwich service for rheumatology. In February 1998 neither the Harrogate Visitors' Centre nor the Town Museum could provide a photograph or postcard depicting the hospital.

Buxton, The Devonshire Royal Hospital

Of the four ex-Spa hospitals, the Devonshire Royal Hospital (DRH) at Buxton was by far and away the most architecturally impressive. The job of Lecturer in Rheumatology at Manchester included a weekly visit to look after the Manchester Royal Infirmary patients who, after investigation in the teaching hospital, were decanted to 30 beds reserved for them for rehabilitation at Buxton. Buxton was about 1000 feet above sea level in the heart of the Peak District. The journey was about 25 miles and could take from about three-quarters of an hour to up to two hours if the weather was bad and the roads were snowed up. Visiting doctors and patients could not help but be struck by the splendour of the place. In the great central arena, covering half an acre and topped by a vast dome, there were in the 1950's and 60's perhaps half a dozen activities going on. A shoulder class in one part. A 'chair rising' class in another. Occupational therapy somewhere else. Perhaps also a snack bar, with chairs put out for a meal. Surrounding this arena were rooms at ground floor and gallery levels. Clinics were held in some of these rooms, physiotherapy in others and the rest were adapted as wards. Beneath it were the hydrotherapy baths fed by the warm spring.

The building had once been the fifth Duke of Devonshire's stables and in 1869 part of the building was presented by the sixth Duke to be a hostel for the sick poor who visited the town for its healing waters. The rest was given in 1881, together with funds to construct the splendid dome.

Dr Ronnie Harris was in charge of rehabilitation. He taught that aids to daily living had to be very simple and preferably made by the patient himself. That way the aids were likely to be valued and used when an 'off the shelf' manufactured gadget would be rejected. He taught the importance of keeping the right balance of ages in the hospital. Elderly patients could be 'psychologically retired' and not easily motivated to rehabilitate themselves. Too many of the old and the morale of the hospital went down for both patients and staff. On the other hand too many young disabled people and there could be a discipline problem. In a hospital such as the Devonshire Royal the sociological aspects of rehabilitation were important. Harris stressed the utility of adaptable uncommitted floor space, a lesson that most hospital planners have yet to learn. The Devonshire Royal Hospital did not confine itself to rheumatism patients but admitted a wide range of rehabilitation problem and disabilities. There was also an active orthopaedic unit. An interesting member of the staff in 1956 was Dr Leo Delicati, as resident Medical Officer, a sort of permanent House Physician previously doing the same job in Bath. He was by then an elderly bachelor, his sole medical qualification was the Licentiate in Medicine and Surgery of the Society of Apothecaries and his one interest outside the hospital was in his annual visit to the meetings of the British Association.

The Lecturer in Rheumatology in 1956 at Manchester and Buxton was Dr Jim Sharp who in 1964 became Consultant to Withington Hospital. His opposite number in Buxton was Dr Stuart Barber, notable for the naming and first comprehensive description of polymyalgia rheumatica. Barber in 1949 had undertaken a small-scale comparison of gold and copper as treatments for rheumatoid arthritis. In contrast to the other Spa hospitals, the Devonshire Royal Hospital took relatively little part in research.

The Hospital was set to close in 1999, if the money could be found to close it. Orthopaedic and rheumatology services were to transfer to the Stepping Hill Hospital where Drs J Marks and P Saunders looked after rheumatology. The reason given was that the orthopaedic patients could not be easily looked after if anything went wrong post-operatively, and that without the orthopaedic contribution, the hospital would not be viable.

Bath, The Royal National Hospital for Rheumatic Diseases.

First called the General Hospital, then in 1826 the Mineral Water Hospital, Bath's spa hospital had been established in 1738 by Beau Nash with charitable subscriptions to be the oldest voluntary hospital outside London. At first it was little more than a 140-bedded hostel to rid the fashionable streets of the sick poor who came to seek relief from their illnesses. Those illnesses were not confined to the rheumatic diseases but included skin problems, 'dropsy', as well as gout from lead poisoning. Gout afflicted painters, shot makers, plumbers, smelters and other lead workers, lead mining and manufacture being a local industry. In 1931 Vincent Coates, a physician to the hospital and Leo Delicati the resident house physician published an analysis of the manifestations of rheumatoid arthritis in 100 consecutive patients (Coates and Delicati, 1931).

The name of the hospital changed in 1936 to The Royal National Hospital for Rheumatic diseases, although it is still known affectionately as the 'Min'. A critical year for the hospital was 1934 when Dr George Kersley was appointed as Physician, having had experience in the Red Cross rheumatism clinic at Peto Place. In 1948 he set up the Rheumatism Research Unit for the Southwest and Oxford Regions, later (1960) supported by the Medical Research Council. Maurice Desmarais, John Dingle and Peter Page-Thomas were among the early researchers. Demarais, with support from Oliver Bird funds, undertook a study of osmic acid injections into osteoarthritic knees and the effects of radiotherapy on rheumatoid joints (with negative results).

Kersley with disarming perseveration would repeatedly describe those years as when the hospital was 'one happy family'. Dr John Cosh, appointed in 1957, recalled that committee members learned to tolerate the 'one happy family' remark whenever it was rehearsed, but privately felt that by then the research had lost momentum.

Kersley had raised funds to rebuild the hospital on a larger site in Bath, plans that were frustrated by the outbreak of war in 1939. He was to see the money disappear when, with the coming of the National Health Service, control passed to the local Hospital Group Management Committee. During the Baedeker air raids the hospital suffered considerable damage and in the 1950's there was doubt as to whether it would continue or whether the site would be sold off. There were those in authority who regarded the hospital as a cuckoo in the nest rather than a jewel in the crown of Bath's medical establishment. Kersley formed a committee that yet again raised funds to rebuild and successfully took his case to the House of Lords. Kersley was unique in that he was the only physician who regularly took his dog, a well-trained alsation, with him on his ward rounds. It was a favourite with the patients but not the senior nursing staff.

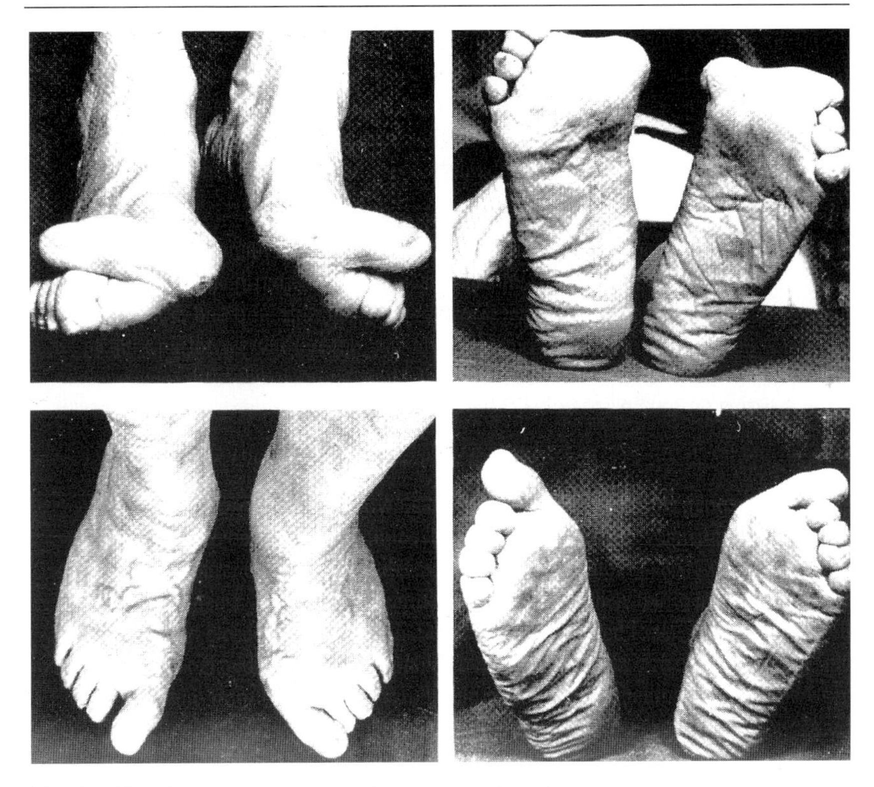

Fig 5.1. The Kates, Kessel, Kay forefoot arthroplasty.

In 1963 the wards and laboratories moved to hutted accommodation in the Royal United Hospital to allow for rebuilding. (Kersley had to be debarred from entering the site as he kept coming up with new suggestions not approved in the plan). In 1965 the refurbished hospital was reopened by Princess Marina, Duchess of Kent with the war damaged parts restored, facilities added which were purpose designed for crippled patients and a new research floor built on top.

The following years were 'golden years' for Bath rheumatology. Older part-time general physicians retired to be replaced by others whose central interest was in the rheumatic diseases. Careful observational studies were made on the eye, heart and other complications of rheumatoid arthritis and ankylosing spondylitis. The surgery of arthritis was explored by John Bastow and later by other orthopaedic colleagues, notably Philip Yeoman, whose father had been the hardworking physician at the Royal Bath Hospital in Harrogate. Combined clinics for hand surgery and for foot surgery were set up.

The psychology of those two clinics was very different. The hand is on show. The hand helps conversation and expresses personality. Patients identify with their hands. Inevitably there is a tendency to operate to improve the appearance of the hand, hoping that improved function will follow. In contrast, feet are hidden. Their owners do not identify with their feet; they only want relief from painful walking. The foot clinic pioneered the use of plaster models of deformed feet, modifying them as lasts on which could be made light-weight comfortable shoes, treating the foot as a packaging problem for a delicate object. Such shoes were very different from the expensive, rigorously defined and heavy surgical shoes previously offered by the National Health Service. When shoes were not practical, because deformities were too severe, patients could be offered operations such as the Kates, Kessell, Kay procedure (Fig 5.1) developed at St Mary Abbots Hospital in Kensington.

This resected the metatarsal heads and replaced the fibro-fatty cushions under the appropriate pressure points. The Bath prosthetic ankle was developed under the pioneering work of John Kirkup. Diabetic and neuropathic foot problems could also be treated, borrowing some of the techniques developed in leprosaria. There seemed more satisfied customers from this clinic than from any other activity of the hospital.

Supernumerary staff were engaged to supervise clinical trials of the new drugs emerging from the drug houses, a 'Robin Hood' activity which helped pay for non-drug research. A series of visiting Fellows mainly from Continental Europe and the Commonwealth countries brought new ideas and doubled the pairs of hands available to undertake research studies.

In 1965, when the hospital had reopened for business after refurbishment, there were three Indian junior doctors with good qualifications. There were problems, however. The Registrar was female and the two male House Physicians were of different castes. Communication between the three was minimal and senior staff who had responsibilities elsewhere could not be sure that all would be looked after their absence.

There is a critical level for the reputation of any hospital. A poor reputation and only the less well motivated apply. A good reputation and good people will want to work there. The struggle was to get on top of that divide. Dr. Julian Kirk, a New Zealander, had been on a Fellowship at Hammersmith but had been dissatisfied with not getting enough 'hands-on' experience. He came to the 'Min' as Registrar and proceeded to build up the standards of junior staff care. An increasing quality of junior staff came to work there and later, when the scheme for Senior House Officer rotations was adopted, it was rare for them not to have the first part of the MRCP examination or the MRCP itself.

The original catchment area for patients was huge; it included Bristol, Exeter, Dorchester, Bournemouth, Swindon and Gloucester. In the late 1960's one quarter of the patients came from South Wales. Bath Spa railway station is on a high level track and special lifts were constructed for the convenience of crippled or wheel chair-bound patients from London, Bristol and South Wales. The lifts ceased to function about 1966 but even by the early 1980's 70% of in-patients came from outside the Bath Clinical Area.

But no hospital exists in an unchanging world. By 1979 it was necessary to ask 'What if?' questions. What if rheumatoid arthritis were found a cure, as had tuberculous arthritis after streptomycin was discovered? What if facilities for rheumatic disease sufferers elsewhere in the Region, which staff at the 'Min' were helping to set up, were such that Bath would no longer be needed? Effective rheumatology services were one by one introduced in the University-linked Bristol Hospitals and in the District General Hospitals throughout the Southwest. Weston-Super-Mare and Barnstaple were the last to be provided for. No longer was the 'Min'; the automatic first choice for rheumatic disease patients or their referring doctors. In 1966 there had been a hospital rule, regularly broken, that patients over 70 would not be admitted. With most younger patients being dealt with in their local hospitals, the 'Min' tended to fill with elderly, complicated or neglected patients who could not be coped with elsewhere. Nothing wrong with that, but as Ronald Harris had taught, it was important to hospital morale, both for patients and staff, to keep a mix of patients representing a spread of ages. The setting up of residential rehabilitation facilities for ankylosing spondylitis sufferers and the appointment of Dr AK Clarke who took on responsibility for paediatric rheumatology helped redress the balance. The ankylosong spondylitis interest has expanded greatly under the direction of Dr Andrei Calin who now has details of over 5000 sufferers, the basis for a number of research and epidemiological studies. Yet there had to be a problem, close to rheumatology, yet unexploited, where the accumulated expertise and resources of the hospital could be put to use. That problem was osteoporosis and in 1986 a special service for osteoporotic patients was inaugurated with the appointment of Dr A Bhalla and Dr Joan Davies as Consultants. This fitted in well with the existing expertise.

Dr John Cosh had initiated the thermography of inflamed joints as a way of measuring the activity of disease and the effect of drugs. The first instrument was a 'Pyroscan' bolometer that gave a reading of the heat flux. In this he was assisted by Mr Francis Ring, at that time a laboratory technician. Cosh also continued his Bristol-acquired interest in cardiology, and was the only physician to be a member both of the British Cardiological Society and of the Heberden Society. This culminated in a scholarly book with John Lever on the cardiac manifestations of rheumatic diseases, published by Springer Verlag in 1986. It did not get much interest from cardiologist colleagues.

Another important achievement was a long-term follow-up of 100 patients seen by Cosh within one year of onset of rheumatoid arthritis. This dated from 1957 and was reviewed in 1973 and at intervals since. Of many findings, one that was particularly striking was the tendency for rheumatoid arthritis to start in the months of December, January and February.

Francis Ring later developed thermographic imaging as improved machines became available, building up an international reputation and a store of knowledge and computer skills that he would later transfer to bone density measurements and osteoporosis. His work and worth were recognised when he was appointed Professor of Medical Physics.

However, osteoporosis is a potentially preventable condition and could disappear. The 'Min' is now developing a Pain Management Unit and diversifying into neuro-rehabilitation which should see it well into the next millennium even if the battles with arthritis and osteoporosis are won.

The Royal National Hospital for Rheumatic Diseases and the University of Bath.

The University of Bath was formed in the late 1960s by the gradual transfer of some parts of the Bristol Polytechnic. It was part of the post-war wave of new universities. Unlike Southampton University, set up at the same time, the faculties did not include an undergraduate medical school despite advocacy by the Professors of Pharmacology and Pharmacy. Their colleagues feared that a medical school in Bath might divert funds from other departments. Neverthrless there was an urge to cooperate with medicine and it pertinent to note the trajectory of one university teacher.

Dr AJ Collins qualified as Ph.D in Pharmacology at the University in 1968. He was interested in inflammatory kinins and was encouraged to submit a proposal to the Research Committee of the Arthritis and Rheumatism Council. At that time the Committee interviewed all applicants. As previously noted, the Committee did not think much of the proposal but did agree to support Collins if he took six months off to learn more about kinins under the expert tuition of Professor Keele of the Middlesex Hospital. This done, Collins returned to Bath and was invited to work in a vacant laboratory in the 'Min', which brought him in contact with the work on thermography and which he exploited as an objective method of quantifying the effects of oral and locally injected anti-inflammatory agents. He found that there was a lag of up to two weeks in the appearance of maximum effects after a non-steroidal anti-inflammatory drug had been given. It also took two weeks when the drug was withdrawn before the effects wore off, a finding that threw doubt on the validity of trials when there was only one week 'wash-out' between the trial drug and comparator.

From 1972 Collins was appointed Lecturer at the University but continued to work with a series of visiting Fellows and Research Registrars at the Hospital. He introduced pharmacy and pharmacology students to clinical ward rounds to improve their understanding of the patients treated by the drugs about which they were learning. In 1976 he was persuaded to train in medicine (by Prof. Jayson). He graduated from Bristol University in 1980 and returned to the 'Min', having learnt the skills of upper gastro-intestinal tract endoscopy. This permitted the direct study of the effects of anti-rheumatic drugs on the lining of the stomach and duodenum. In 1986 he discovered a new spiral micro-organism resident in the duodenum.

By the late 1970s the University of Bath had shown itself favourable to closer links with the hospital system, attracted by the considerable research that was taking place there. At first the lion's share of this was conducted at the 'Min' often by cooperative efforts between its personnel and those of the University. Medically related research also increased in other parts of the hospital group starting with the appointment of Professor Lillycrap in Medical Physics, two physicians as Honorary Lecturers, and two as Visiting Professors. A series of semi-independent medical research institutes affiliated to the University were set up. They catered for medical engineering, paediatrics, care of the elderly and the rheumatic diseases.

The Bath Institute for Rheumatic Diseases.

Another 'what if' question inspired the development of the Bath Institute for Rheumatic Diseases: 'what would happen if funds for the Hospital's research programme were to dry up?

About 1975 the government altered the law so that donations to universities (but not to NHS hospitals) would be tax free to the donor. Technically, the 'Min' was a NHS non-teaching hospital. As such it could not receive tax-free donations, although it produced more research papers than the rest of Bath hospitals put together and had regular teaching sessions for Bristol undergraduates. This stimulated the setting up of an independent Research Institute, which would handle research funding and charitable donations and which would be affiliated to the University of Bath. In 1983, funds were raised to buy and re-equip as research laboratories a vacant printing works opposite the hospital. Soon the research output was such that Bath University took more notice and by 1985 agreed to set up a Postgraduate School of Medicine. Dr. Peter Maddison of the 'Min' was appointed Glaxo Professor of Osteoarticular Medicine and Dean.

Recent Developments

Why did the Royal National Hospital for Rheumatic Diseases in Bath survive when two of the other three spa hospitals had died and the third was scheduled for closure? Much of the credit for masterminding its survival must go to Dr AK (Tony) Clarke.

Dr Clarke was appointed to the 'Min ' on Sept. 1st 1977 around the time of the closing of the civic spa facilities. His appointment arose from the need for rehabilitation expertise emphasised by the DHSS Working Party set up under the ministry of Sir Keith Joseph. Clarke's previous experience had been with John Goodwill, at King's College Hospital, who in turn had trained under Frank Cooksey. Unlike most doctors, Clarke had a liking for committee work and administration, qualities that fitted him to face the battles for the future of the 'Min' and to midwife the necessary adaptations under the NHS reforms.

In 1990 when the National Health Service and Community Care act came in, it promised to streamline the Regional and District Health Authorities and Family Health Service and to establish NHS Trusts which would operate as self governing health care 'providers'. Family doctors who needed to call in hospital services would be the 'purchasers' and would be in contract with the providers. From the first of April 1992 Community Care reforms changed the way care was delivered to the handicapped and elderly. Regional Offices that would monitor health care provision but would not have direct administrative powers replaced Regional Health Authorities.

When the National Health Service had been inaugurated in 1948, the 'Min' had been a semi-independent entity under its own Management Committee, with finance provided from the Region. But under successive Health Service reforms it had gradually lost autonomy to the Bath Health District Administration located in the Royal United Hospital (RUH). The original Management Committee, which had been comprised of local persons of good will, had been abolished under the 'Cogwheel' reforms. Despite its national status and name, the Royal National Hospital for Rheumatic Diseases enjoyed the administrative status of a cottage hospital governed by absentee landlords. All radiology, laboratory, and building maintenance services that had once been provided in house had now to be requested from the RUH site, entailing delays and paper work. Originally Bath Health District had looked to Avon for its Regional administration and to Bristol University Medical School for input into staff appointments. Under the reforms this changed to Wessex and Southampton, opening a gap between Bath and those Bristol rheumatology services that traditionally had been linked to Bath. The valuable but inconvenient city centre site of the 'Min' was again considered for sale and the hospital for relocation. By 1990 sites had been inspected and plans advanced. The individuality and history of the hospital were threatened, however, and no one was in a hurry to move.

When in 1992 the government White Paper on the restructuring of the Health Service was announced on the radio at 2 pm, applications were invited to join the first wave of hospital trusts. By 4 PM on that day Tony Clarke and Clive Quinnel, the hospital Administrator, had requested the necessary papers. The dash for Trust status was on.

The 'Min' joined in the first wave, ahead of the other Bath hospitals, thus repossessing control of its future. Its status as an academic specialist teaching hospital, part of the Bath University, was assured. Colleagues in the other hospitals who still thought that the Min was non-viable and should be sold off to benefit general funds were too late.

How long, nevertheless, could it continue? Trust status had enabled extensive internal restructuring. With fewer rheumatoid arthritis patients flocking to the hospital there was a need for diversification. The hospital's original operating theatre, long since vacated by the surgeons, developed an endoscopy unit, combining research into the gastrointestinal effects of anti-rheumatic drugs and their antidotes with an efficient service for family doctors. Half of the beds were redesignated for neuro-rehabiltation. The osteoporosis service prospered and the hospital was solvent. Between 1989 and 1997 the hospital's annual financial turnover rose from £4 1/2 m to £8 1/2m.

The first possible threat to these changes came when the Gwent Health Authority decided to rationalise its services. They had too many rheumatology service providers, of which the 'Min' was one. It was decided to put in a joint bid with the Nevil Hall Hospital to provide all the services. Either that or go bankrupt. The bid was accepted. At Neath there was a waiting list of 400 rheumatology referrals. Some patients had waited four years. Dr Tom Jenkinson was sent for a week to work off the list and Drs A Clarke and L Clarke visited once a month. Dr Nigel Cox at Winchester was faced with a problem of providing a service for Andover and linking to the 'Min' solved that.

It was foreseen that, if there were to be a rearrangement of health service boundaries, the 'Min' would link with Southmead Hospital. Bristol rheumatology services would be consolidated there.

In 1989 the 'Min' celebrated its first quarter millennium. Would it see a second?

Chapter 6
Rheumatology in the District General Hospitals
Three Exemplary Centres

In 1992 the journal *Hospital Doctor* hit upon a scheme for a competition between specialist hospital services for the title of 'Hospital Doctor of the Year'. Many specialties of medicine were represented, such as Cardiology Hospital Doctor of the year, Geriatrics Hospital Doctor of the year etc. Amongst these were Rheumatology Hospital Doctor of the Year and Osteoporosis Hospital Doctor of the Year. The judging criteria (summarised) were:

1. Effective team working.
2. Involvement and communication with patients.
3. Innovation and new ways of working.
4. Is the doctor the driving force for change?
5. How well is the team doing in the setting it finds itself?

The winners could claim kudos but more importantly a sum of money to improve their services. Each title was sponsored by a drug company. There were large numbers of entries from which, for each speciality, three hospital teams would be short-listed and one would be the eventual winner.

The 'Rheumatology Hospital Doctor of the Year' team winners were:

1992 Freeman Hospital in Newcastle,
1993 Christchurch Hospital in Dorset,
1994 Huddersfield Hospital in West Yorkshire,
1995 Cannock Chase Hospital in Staffordshire,
1996 South Cleveland Hospital in Middlesbrough,
1997 Norfolk and Norwich Hospital in Norwich.

There were twelve runners up. Together they exemplified the progress made in District General Hospitals in the last 50 years. Three examples illustrate that progress.

Norfolk and Norwich Hospital. Prof. DGI Scott's team

In 1948 and until 1959 there were no specialist services for rheumatism sufferers among the two million population of East Anglia. In Cambridge Dr Fell (Physical Medicine) had expressed no interest and rheumatic diseases were treated by general physicians. Orthopaedic surgeons operated on the more severely disabled.

Dr DGI Scott qualified in Bristol in 1973 and after training posts in Bristol, Bath and Birmingham had been appointed Consultant in Rheumatology to the Norfolk and Norwich Hospital on February 1st 1988. Ten years later, building on the excellent service given to rheumatology patients by his predecessors, David Scott and his team entered for and won the title of '1997 Rheumatology Hospital Doctor of the Year'.

His special interest was vasculitis. With his colleague Peter Merry he inherited a comprehensive rheumatology service with a fine reputation for service. This had been the achievement of Dr Neil Cardoe who had been Registrar at the Arthur Stanley Institute (the successor of the Red Cross Clinic at Peto Place). Cardoe had been appointed in October 1959 as General Physician with an interest in the rheumatic diseases to the Norfolk and Norwich, Cromer, Kelling Children's and Mundesley Hospitals. Great Yarmouth Hospital and various cottage hospitals were added at a later date. He held clinics once or twice a week at the main hospitals and looked after 60 in-patient beds.

St Michael's Hospital at Aylsham where he was to develop a rheumatology service had been built in 1848 as a poor law hospital. The punishment cells and lime closets still existed a hundred years later. The wards, heated by coke stoves, had wooden floors that tended to splinter. A small side ward housed physiotherapy. There were neither X-ray nor pathology facilities.

Things changed rapidly. By November 1960 there were 30 rheumatology beds at Aylsham, an occupational therapy department and enlarged physiotherapy departments. The old laundry had been converted into a hydrotherapy pool and beds were added to a total of 48. An X-ray department had been built and pathology services made available. In 1962 a gift of £1,500 from the Hirst family helped equip an orthopaedic operating theatre.

The Regional Hospital Board, in response to the increasing workload, planned to appoint two rheumatology or rehabilitation specialists in each of the four sub regions of East Anglia. Dr Gil Wenley joined him in 1964. Appointments at Peterborough, Cambridge, Ipswich and Bury St. Edmunds soon followed. Dr John Burrows in 1966 built up the rehabilitation services. Soon a comprehensive regional service was in being.

In 1973 Dr Cardoe gave the Heberden Round on the theme of general medicine and rheumatology. That year Norwich, Aylsham and Mundesley hospitals were named by the DHSS as centres of excellence and allocated £100,000 to upgrade facilities. At Aylsham three wards were further improved and new and fully equipped physiotherapy and occupational therapy departments provided. Workshop and physiotherapy amenities were upgraded at Mundesley. The Norfolk and Norwich Hospital needed only minor changes as the Duchess of Kent had recently opened a completely new department.

Nevertheless surgical facilities at Aylsham were inadequate and there were long waiting lists. In 1980 a gala performance at the Norwich Theatre Royal in the presence of the Duchess of Kent helped raise £450,000 to build a dedicated arthritis operating theatre. This was completed in 1981 and by 1982 there were almost daily operating sessions. No emergency care was carried out so surgeons were able to operate without accident cases interrupting their work. In 1980 combined out-patient clinics were started with orthopaedic surgeons and paediatricians. Kelling Children's Hospital was briefly a regional paediatric rheumatology centre. It was closed in 1966 and the work transferred to Aylsham.

Before Dr Scott arrived in 1988 research and teaching were less developed. Changes, however, were on the way. After 1991 Aylsham progressively lost its medical services. Because of worries about proper care for emergencies complicating surgery, operations were transferred to other hospitals. By 1998 there were five regular clinics shared between rheumatologists and individual 'upper limb' or 'lower limb' orthopaedic surgeons, although all do hip replacements. One surgeon, Hugh Philips, was to be the next President of the British Orthopaedic Association.

Norwich's orthopaedic tradition had been built on the pioneering work of Ken McKee and his hip arthroplasty. (When McKee was chairman of the Medical Committee he insisted that its deliberations should always start with a short prayer meeting.)

Paediatric rheumatology was served by a two-weekly clinic shared with paediatrician Marc Dyke and by a six monthly visit from Prof T. Southwood from Birmingham, useful to help confidence with rarer conditions such as neonatal sarcoidosis. There was no adolescent rheumatology service and this was recognised to be a deficiency. Nor was there an osteoporosis service although the rheumatologists could call on the help of Philip Heyburn, bone disease specialist and the NHS Trust would pay for up to 300 DXA bone scans each year in the local private hospital.

The rheumatology department at the Norfolk and Norwich Hospital was the base for a primary care nurse-staffed telephone help line and for nurse practitioner clinics where treatments such as gold or methotrexate could be monitored. It contained a Day Unit, estimated to save £300,000 a year by enabling inpatient bed closures. An early arthritis clinic provided a fast track referral service. Patients' advice had been incorporated into every aspect of the team's work.

By 1992 Aylsham had closed as a hospital, surviving only as the base for the Norfolk Arthritis Register 'NOAR', the brainchild of Alan Silman and Deborah Symmons of the ARC Epidemiology unit in Manchester. Its loss did not seem to have evoked the sense of betrayal that others have experienced when they had seen their life's work dismantled, perhaps because of the promise of more and better to come. NOAR was locally managed by Bett Barrett with ARC funding and had six other staff, including five metrologists who visited patients in their homes, doctors' surgeries or in one of the hospitals. All NOAR-registered patients had serum and gene DNA stored. NOAR had already shown that the incidence of rheumatoid arthritis rose with age in men, and that involvement of the knees was associated with a poor prognosis. A case/control study which started in 1994 (Simmons et al, 1997) showed that obesity, smoking and previous blood transfusions were positive risk factors for rheumatoid arthritis. A local group planned to use the database to study the prevalence in the East Anglian population of the HLA-H gene mutation known to be associated with haemochromatosis, with the object of finding hidden cases.

David GI Scott was Professor in the University of East Anglia at Norwich. There was co-operation with the School of Health in the University with the appointment of Maria Koutanji, non-clinical psychologist, as an ARC-funded lecturer. The University ran a successful course leading to MSc in Health Science and as part of this Scott and a lecturer in Occupational Therapy were organising a module in rheumatic diseases.

The Norfolk and Norwich Hospital was scheduled to move in 2002 to a green field site next to the University of East Anglia, funded by private finance initiative money. The academic activities of the rheumatology group were expected to expand.

Prof. Ian Haslock's team at the South Cleveland Hospital, Middlesbrough, winners in 1996

In 1948, as in East Anglia, services for arthritis sufferers in Teeside were virtually non-existent. It fell to Dr Desmond Newton to change all that.

Desmond Newton was born in 1922. He was a wartime St Thomas's student qualifying in 1945 before military service took him to India and Japan. He returned to St Thomas's Hospital for postgraduate training and became Chief Assistant to the Department of Physical Medicine at St Thomas's until 1959 when he was appointed as Consultant Physician (Rheumatology and Rehabilitation) to North and South Teeside, Darlington and Northallerton hospitals. There he set up a physiotherapy service and later a school of physiotherapy.

He was a respected and painstaking diagnostician with a clear and logical mind, much in demand also for work on committees. He was important in the evolution of rheumatology and its separation from rehabilitation. He served on the governing bodies of the Section of Physical Medicine of the Royal Society of Medicine, the British Association for Rheumatology and Rehabilitation and the Joint Committee for Higher Medical Training of the Royal College of Physicians. He was Chairman of its Specialist Advisory Committee on Rheumatology 1974 to 1976.

In 1965 Newton opened the first specialist rheumatology ward in the Northern Region and in 1972 he appointed the Region's first specialist rheumatology out-patient nurse. He retired in 1987.

In 1973 Dr Ian Haslock joined him as second Consultant Rheumatologist. Haslock had qualified in 1965 at Leeds and worked at the Royal Bath Hospital in Harrogate when he came to the notice of the late Prof Verna Wright. Wright invited Haslock to become his Registrar in rheumatology at Leeds General Hospital. There Haslock became interested in two of Wright's special concerns, bioengineering and enteropathic arthritis. The latter was to be the subject of his MD thesis.

Once at South Cleveland, Haslock set about tackling all aspects of rheumatology. This entailed innovative work with nurses and other health professionals leading to the team winning the title of Rheumatology Hospital of the Year in 1996.

Dr John Fordham who had qualified in 1972 and had been Senior Registrar in Rheumatology at the London Hospital had joined him in 1984.

When Haslock was appointed to the Consultant job in Middlesbrough General Hospital in 1973 he worked alongside Newton and their offices and out-patient clinics were still in the Physiotherapy department. Later beds became available at the West Lane Hospital for Infectious Diseases in wards with open balconies originally designed for tuberculosis patients. When that hospital closed, beds were moved to

Hemlington Hospital, an old wartime Emergency Medical Services hospital. A new block for rheumatology was built at South Cleveland Hospital in exchange for the closing of Hemlington.

The unit was strong in surgical Rheumatology and was running a number of combined orthopaedic / rheumatology clinics. Thus Haslock did a hand clinic with plastic surgeon Charles Viva, an upper limb clinic with orthopaedic surgeon John Stothard, and another with orthopaedic surgeon John Anderson. Fordham undertook a hand and upper limb clinic with John Stothard and also a clinic with orthopaedic surgeon Ian Wallace. The system of involving two consultants was admittedly expensive in consultant time, but the payback for the surgeons was that the patients were already screened as suitable.

Fordham's special interest was in osteoporosis and he was instrumental in winning the title of Osteoporosis Hospital Doctor of the Year for his team in 1996 – two successes in one year for the hospital. In 1997 Fordham became a member of the Council of Management of the National Osteoporosis Society.

Dr Fiona Clarke with Dr Myint Oo, paediatric consultant, shared paediatric rheumatology in Tees Side. It was planned to start an adolescent rheumatology service.

South Cleveland Hospital looked to three universities for its academic links:

1. Tees Side University. This was developing a School of Health Sciences, a School of Physiotherapy, and a School of Occupational Therapy. It awarded a MSc in clinical orthopaedics and a MSc in ultrasound. It was strong in information technology.

2. Durham University, which might soon get a preclinical school. Haslock was a Visiting Professor in Clinical Bioengineering at Durham University.

3. Newcastle University, which sent undergraduates for experience and training at Middlesbrough.

Advances were being made in the radiology of rheumatic diseases. One radiologist had been appointed specially to look after ultrasound techniques and was studying soft tissue lesions around the shoulder tendons and neck. Nuclear magnetic resonance had supplanted an open access arthroscopy service. It was more informative for knees, neck and lumbar spine.A computer system that had been installed in the rheumatology department at South Cleveland Hospital saved an enormous amount of time in record keeping. A practising rheumatologist had written its software, so it was user-friendly.

Recently Haslock had become Medical Director of the hospital. He was President of the British Society for Rheumatology in 1988 after it was formed by the fusion of the Heberden Society and the British Society for Rheumatology and Rehabilitation in 1984. He was also President of the British League against Rheumatism, the organisation charged with hosting the European League against Rheumatism at its congress in Glasgow in 1999.

Truro, The Duke of Cornwall Rheumatism Unit. Team leader Dr AD Woolf

The third unit chosen was one of the three finalists in 1996 although not the winner. The Duke of Cornwall Rheumatism Unit in Truro served a population of 475,000 in the county of Cornwall and the Isles of Scilly apart from those bits that were closer to hospitals in Barnstaple and Plymouth. Like the other two exemplary services, it had come up from nothing in the last 50 years but unlike them the first phase of its existence, even the building in which it was housed, reflected the efforts of one individual. A '*Medical Directory*' citation might read:

Thould, Anthony Keith, *MD Lond. 1960 (by thesis on the association of congenital goitre and high tone deafness), FRCP 1974, Gilliland Fellowship 1983, Surg Lt. Commander RNR, Editor of the Annals of Rheumatic Diseases 1988, ex Bart's Senior Registrar in Rheumatology and ex-University College Hospital Registrar in Medicine. Papers on Arthritis in Roman Britain (jointly with his manciple), Constrictive Pericarditis in Rheumatoid Arthritis, Computers in Rheumatology, the 'Exit Syndrome', Xray aspects of rheumatoid joint erosions, etc.*

When in 1965 Thould was appointed to Truro Hospitals as Consultant Physician, medicine was practiced as in the 1940's. On arrival Thould was forbidden to set up a rheumatism clinic despite his experience in rheumatology. Instead he established a coronary care unit and a service for continuous ambulatory peritoneal dialysis. This fitted in with the gradual development of the (then) new Treliske hospital, the first phase of which opened a few months after his appointment. Under his general medical hat he reported on the incidence of heart attacks in car drivers over-stressed during the summer lemming-like holiday rush from the Midlands to Cornwall.

Rheumatology did not exist in Cornwall in 1965; a state of affairs that continued unchanged until the early 1970's. An older physician oversaw a physiotherapy service with a few beds in an ex-workhouse Hospital. "He didn't know what he was doing in rheumatology", (Thould's opinion) and "was using massive and indiscriminate doses of corticosteroids."

By 1970 something had to be done about the rheumatology service. The population was aging and rheumatic diseases more prevalent. His proposals for doing that something were opposed by his colleagues and he was offered a derisory twelve beds in a converted ward in Tehidy Hospital, where there would have been no physiotherapy department, an inadequate Xray service and no orthopaedic input.

It was a make or break stage and colleagues were told that a proper rheumatism unit had to be provided for the people of Cornwall, 'whether you like it or not'. In this he received support from Belinda Balham, the forward-looking Chairman of the SouthWest Regional Hospital Board. Told to choose between Treliske, the City and Tehidy Hospitals, he chose the City site, because of the then association with the orthopaedic services. One physician had written to the Regional Medical Officer demanding that 'this must be stopped'. Luckily no notice was taken. The hospital authorities granted £100,000 and Thould was encouraged to raise further funds him self. In 1974 an appeal was launched with Lady Falmouth as the indefatigable Chairman. £250,000 was raised as a result of going the rounds of Rotary Clubs, Women's Institutes and public Charities during two hectic years with scarcely ever an evening at home. Marion Smith, his secretary, recorded that some 23,000 letters had been written during the campaign. Drs and Professors Barbara Ansell, at Taplow, Eric Bywaters at Hammersmith, George Kersley at Bath and Jonas Kellgren at Manchester had provided ideas to be incorporated into the design of the Unit. With this money in hand the accountant was able to advise a building start. In 1978 the Prince of Wales opened the first phase of the new Duke of Cornwall Rheumatism Unit. It provided 12 beds and out-patients clinics, its own plaster room, physiotherapy and occupational therapy services and a day area so that patients were not confined to their wards. Money was tight: At first only eight of the twelve beds could be opened. (The empty beds were kept on show as a reminder to visitors that more funds were still needed).

Under the stimulus of one of his patients, Alice Barbario, Thould decided to raise money for a second floor. There was no problem about the foundations as these had been designed with forethought to take the extra weight. A further £250,000 was raised and in 1980 the Duchess of Gloucester opened the new floor. The completed building was the first purpose-designed rheumatology unit in England. It housed offices for the staff, a medical library, a lecture room and space for research facilities as well as the beds and outpatients' treatment areas.

Thould's rheumatology team called themselves the 'Truro Salvage Corps', their first job to get on top of the load of untreated, mistreated and often derelict rheumatoid arthritis patients and to wean those who were on it off over-treatment with corticosteroids. Two Community Liaison nurses were appointed. They would keep in touch with patients in their own homes. Twice a week ward rounds were followed by a team conference.

A children's rheumatism clinic followed (despite opposition from paediatric and nursing services), and a hemophilia arthritis service, (with enthusiastic support from the haematologists). Once the bleeding tendency was under control it was possible to undertake knee replacements and other operations for the haemophiliacs. An Ankylosing Spondylitis service, with advice from Bath physiotherapist Sarah Barton, and a foot clinic were started on the Bath models. A combined medical and surgical rheumatology clinic was planned but did not prosper, nevertheless the battle for new hips for arthritis patients was engaged and won, but failure to get knee replacements for those who needed them was distressing.

Inevitably there were accusations of 'Empire Building' and the case for every new development had to be made out in statistically supported detail. A diagnostic index was essential in order to keep a tally of the different diagnoses and patients. Thould applied for and was awarded a BMA-Gilliland Fellowship to visit Stanford University in California to see how subjects and events were documented in their Coronary Prevention Service. Further ideas came from Bethesda and the Massachusetts General Hospital.

Working as a single-handed consultant in a peripheral hospital had advantages and disadvantages. There was a need for support from colleagues, especially when the successful fund-raising generated envy and enmity among some of them. On the other hand there was no danger of the clashes of personality that can arise when two or more consultants share the same field of interest. Thould admitted that he took strong likes (for example to Prof. Max Rosenheim) and dislikes (to Prof. Scowen). He also expressed affection for Dr Wykeham Balme, his consultant at St Bartholomew's.

For other professional contacts it had been helpful to talk with Drs. Richard Jacoby, Consultant Rheumatologist at Torbay, and David Yates at Taunton and to have occasional visits by the author from Bath. To extend these contacts an unofficial Regional Rheumatology Advisory Committee was set up, to include all the rheumatology services in the SouthWest as they came into being. Through this Advisory Committee Thould worked successfully for the appointment of a consultant rheumatologist in all but two of the District General Hospitals in the SouthWest.[8] Three years before Thould's retirement, Dr AD Woolf joined him from Bristol.

Relationships with rehabilitation services were not a problem, unlike the experience in some London Hospitals. His colleague rehabilitation specialist was Dr Chris Evans who had been Services-trained had a separate office and a different orbit of interest.

Thould became concerned about the relative lack of attention paid by rheumatologists to the problem of osteoarthitis. He set up an annual meeting the proceedings of which were called the 'Pendragon Papers,' a multidisciplinary forum that met and discussed this common and neglected condition. Three meetings were held, later discontinued for lack of funds. He also had a pivotal influence in convincing the Arthritis and Rheumatism Council that it should set up a Chair of Rheumatology in Bristol with the primary target of osteoarthritis. He asked Dr Paul Dieppe to consider applying for the Senior Lecturer position in Bristol following Dr Malcolm Jayson. An appointments committee was selected. In the event an application from Dieppe was not received until well after the published deadline but could be accepted because this was an academic, not a National Health Service, appointment.

Thould's work did not ease up after Dr Woolf's appointment. He accepted to be Editor of the 'Annals of Rheumatic Diseases' a busy and stressful job. This led to an event that decided him to retire early on health grounds.

The local Health Executive then delivered a distressing blow. It decided that the City Hospital would be closed and all the services including rheumatology moved to the Treliske site. Pleas to retain the Rheumatism Unit's building as a Rehabilitation Centre for the whole of Cornwall fell on deaf ears. This destruction of much that he had striven for was felt as a betrayal.

He need not have worried. His successor Dr AD Woolf saw this as an opportunity to make further improvements in the service. His Medical Directory might read:

Woolf, Anthony Derek, *MRCP (London), qualified from the London Hospital in 1975, previously Senior Registrar at the Royal National Hospital for Rheumatic Diseases in Bath and the Bristol Royal Infirmary and Registrar in General Medicine and Rheumatology at Guy's Hospital. Joint author of 'Osteoporosis-A Clinical Guide' and papers on osteoporosis and viral arthritis. Chairman of the National Osteoporosis Society.*

8 At Barnstaple and Weston-Super-Mare. Consultants services were provided there later.

Dr Woolf would have been well aware of what he was getting into when he chose to become a rheumatologist. He was the son of Douglas Woolf, previously rheumatologist at the Willesden and Central Middlesex Hospitals and Chairman of Arthritis Care.

In the move from Bristol he inherited a purpose-built rheumatology unit and after Thould's retirement was joined by Dr Martin Davis, consultant. The team's approach to community rheumatology was strengthened further so that patients with chronic rheumatic diseases could be assured of continuing support, a 'hub and spokes' approach to shared care between specialist unit and family doctors pioneered by his predecessor. Parenthetically this differed from the hub and spokes philosophy practiced in Edinburgh, where the hub was the university hospital to which all rheumatologists were appointed and the spokes the peripheral hospitals where they mainly worked. In Cornwall peripheral clinics were held in some of the many small hospitals in the County. The specialist nurses educated the GPs' practice nurses about the management of rheumatic disorders and visited the patients on discharge. They reported back on any domestic or other factors that might affect the patient's progress. A comment from a patient was: 'These people know us, are supporting us, this is great'

Further community liaison was through the local branch of the British League against Rheumatism (BLAR) which could also act as an 'umbrella' organisation for disability research and self-help groups[9] and a lever against administrative attempts to reduce beds and facilities. The 18 dedicated beds in the unit had already been reduced to 14 and there were threats of reduction to 10 five-day beds on the planned move to the Treliske site. Woolf believed that beds were essential in a widely scattered population such as Cornwall where there was only one rheumatology service for the county.

The early rheumatoid arthritis sufferer was admitted early and received a full medical examination and appropriate investigations, an explanation of the disease and treatment proposed and introduction to the community nurses who were to maintain contact after discharge. In addition to educating the patient and her carer, the nurse assessed attitudes and the home environment. "You don't want to start treating a patient with methotrexate because she complains of getting worse, if the real problem is a family one."

Chiropody and careful shoe prescriptions have been emphasised. "We hardly ever do ankle injections or metatarsal arthroplasties". An open access telephone help line run by the community nurses had a separate British Telecom line, an answer phone and a mobile phone for when the nurse was away from base. "If you are trying to keep the numbers admitted to hospital as low as possible, the ones discharged are by definition almost as bad as those that are still in. It's daft not to know what's happening to them" A 'rheumatoid arthritis log book' was planned to act as the patient's own record of treatments, appointments and disease events.

A survey by an Occupational Therapist noted that while the needs of the severely disabled were usually met and those with mild disability were coping, it was

9 Arthritis Research Campaign, Arthritis Care, National Ankylosing Spondylitis Society, National Osteoporosis Society, etc.

the 'middle-ground' severity of patients with rheumatoid arthritis who were ignored unless routinely assessed.

In an initiative sponsored by Searle there had been appointed selected 'Patient Partners' who helped teach trainee medical staff how to take a rheumatological history and do a rheumatological examination. Dr. Elaine Hay, appointed in Stoke on Trent as the first consultant Community Rheumatologist in England, was following much the same approach.

Woolf was not too alarmed by the prospect of closure of the Unit and the transfer to Treliske in 1999. In the event he was given the facilities to do the job properly and there were advantages to being a unit within the District General Hospital. Critical to his thinking was the provision of a large, multi-purpose day room, an open space where many activities and meetings could take place. Public meetings would be open and would deal with topics like 'How to cope', 'Self care', and 'Recent research'.

The Rheumatism Unit is currently one of only two services in the Truro hospitals regularly undertaking research and it is beginning to collaborate with Plymouth University where Woolf has been awarded a personal Chair. Until this develops further, Prof Woolf will continue research 'net-working' with Manchester (Prof Alan Silman), King's College Hospital and Bath.

Some conclusions

All three services had built on the pioneering efforts of their predecessors and all three were developing university links that were likely to become more important. Specialist nurses were ensuring the delivery of rheumatology care to those who required it but some fully staffed beds were essential for rheumatism units to do their work. This would have to be emphasised at national level as severe rheumatoid arthritis could present some of the most challenging problems to medical and nursing services. The advent of local injection therapy for arthritis and stronger drugs such as methotrexate had reduced but not removed the need for beds. There needed to be a greater understanding on the part of the administrators of the support required for the hospital-based team approach to community care. District general hospitals were likely to be better placed than teaching hospitals to deliver community care rheumatology.

There will be an ever-increasing contribution from information technology. Rheumatology departments can link through Medline to half the world's literature to support the publications and teaching material they issue. Specialist nurses will take on more responsibilities and in turn will need certification of their capabilities.

Chapter 7
Paediatric Rheumatology

Few can now recall the scourge of rheumatic fever and rheumatic heart disease in the first part of this century, affecting every country and especially the urban poor although the children of the well to do were not exempt. In London alone thousands of beds in paediatric wards, fever hospitals and convalescent homes were set aside for the victims of rheumatic fever, according to a survey by Francis Bach and his colleagues, published in the first issue of the Annals of Rheumatic Diseases. (Bach et al., 1939). The incidence had been slowly declining with improvements in living standards but with the crowding together of children in wartime dormitories and bomb-shelters numbers would have risen. Rheumatic fever became of military significance when young men were herded into training camps and cramped ships. As trained recruits moved on, new recruits with little immunity took their place. The causative microorganism was 'passaged' and virulence built up. After the armistice rheumatic fever was still rife in the UK and the USA.

'Rheumatic fever licks the joints but bites the heart'. Three per cent of all streptococcal throat infections in children were followed by rheumatic fever and of these twenty per cent would suffer permanent heart damage. Rheumatic fever was recurrent, according to whether there was further infection. Twenty per cent of those with residual heart damage would die within 20 years. To this toll would be added those young adults who presented with rheumatic heart disease never having had overt rheumatic fever. In this climate Still's Disease, as chronic arthritis in children was then called, received less attention.

That rheumatic fever had a bacterial cause and that the cause was a streptococcus was widely accepted but unproved before the war (Wilson, 1940) The significance of the different Lancefield streptococcal groups and Griffiths types was not fully realised. It was the pioneering epidemiological work of Rammelkamp in Detroit that confirmed the association, finally proved by the ability of antibiotics to prevent recurrence of the disease.

The Canadian Red Cross Memorial Hospital was built at Taplow in the grounds of Lady Astor's property at Cliveden for the Canadian forces during the Second World War (Figure 7.1). It was offered to the UK Government at the end of it with the wish that it should be used for research into rheumatism in children (Bywaters, 1998). It had accommodation for about 600 beds, mostly in hutted 'Nightingale' type 30-bedded wards. A hospital that only admitted rheumatic children was impracticable. Instead it was set up as a working general hospital with medical, surgical, chest, obstetric, and 'non-rheumatic' children's units so that a full range of consultant expertise would be available for a large Special Unit for Juvenile Rheumatism. This had 75 beds in three wards, with another ward adapted as research laboratories. Dr Eric Bywaters, then a lecturer at Hammersmith Hospital, British Postgraduate Medical School (BPMS), had had pre-war experience of rheumatoid arthritis and systemic lupus, and had done pioneering wartime work on the crush syndrome. He was appointed to the Special Unit as Director, but continuing his attachment to the BPMS. It was a brilliant appointment. It would be hard to see something similar happening with today's more rigid

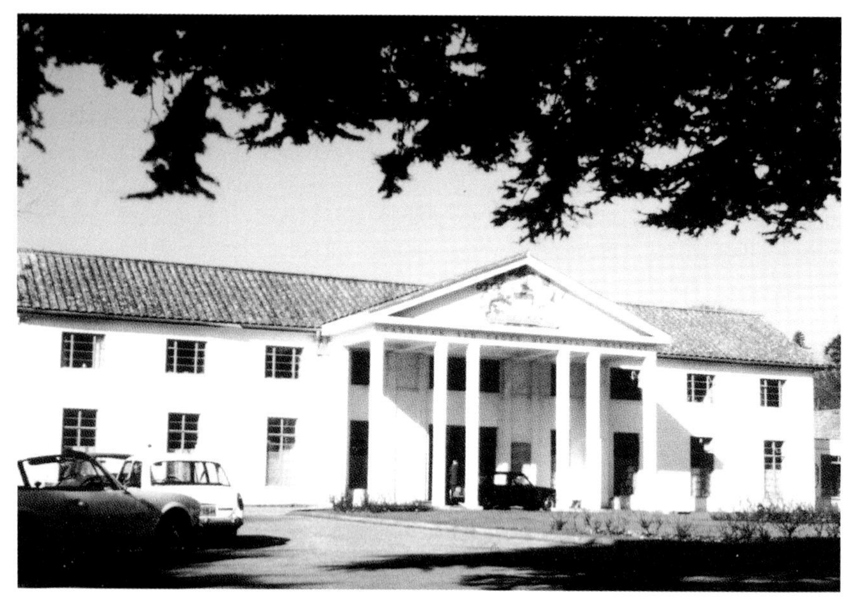

Fig 7.1. The Canadian Red Cross Memorial Hospital.

demarcation of medical specialities. Rheumatic fever was a disease of children and of children's hearts. The new director had little in his *curriculum vitae* to say that he had special experience either in paediatrics or cardiology.

Bywaters first move after appointment was to make a prolonged tour of all the important rheumatologists and rheumatology centres in the USA and Canada, particularly those that specialised in rheumatic fever. One was the House of the Good Samaritan under the direction of T. Ducket Jones, who defined the widely adopted criteria for the diagnosis of rheumatic fever (Bywaters, 1949). The hospital was opened for business in 1947 and the wards were soon full. Cardiological expertise was supplied by Dr. Gerald Thomas and by weekly visits by Dr Paul Wood from the National Heart Hospital. The staff eagerly awaited Paul Wood's visits. He had brought examination and auscultation of the cardiovascular system in children to a fine art, building on the work of Carey Coombs (Coombs, 1924) with the added advantage of knowledge gained at open heart surgery. Dr Reggie Lightwood from Great Ormond Street Hospital advised on paediatric issues. There were four registrars to look after the wards and run follow-up out-patient clinics in the National Heart, Hammersmith, Isleworth, Slough and Reading Hospitals. They were also responsible, along with visiting Fellows and the staff of the Research laboratory under Dr LE Glynn, as pairs of hands to promote the research projects. Everything had to be measured. One of the registrars, Dr Madeline Keech, tried hypnosis to see if she could reduce the abnormal movements in chorea, and there was a 'chorea bed' designed to summate and quantify the movements that a child would make at night. There was a sound proofed phonocardiography room to record heart sounds and a primitive ballistocardiograph to measure aortic reflux.

Treatment was by bed rest and aspirin, with antibiotics to clear residual throat infection. This was followed by chemoprophylaxis with injections of benzathine penicillin or tablets of a sulphonamide to prevent reinfection and recurrences. Bed rest was later modified when it found that there was less strain on the heart sitting up than when supine. Aspirin was given in large doses, monitored by salicylate blood levels. Even so aspirin toxicity was common, with vomiting, deafness, tinnitus and occasionally more serious problems of fluid retention in children with heart failure. Aspirin makes feverish children sweat copiously. Traditionally children were nursed in blankets because of this, but the tradition was soon abandoned in Taplow. In 1949 there was conversation between Bywaters and Lightwood concerning the original purpose of the Special Unit and whether children with Still's disease should be admitted, as they might not fit in with the routines established for rheumatic fever. It was an early decision that they should.

In 1950 the Special Unit took part in the US-UK multicentre controlled trial of aspirin, cortisone and ACTH in rheumatic fever, advised by medical statisticians Prof. Austin Bradford Hill and Dr John Knowelden. The Medical Research Council appointed the author as registrar to visit UK co-operating hospitals to ensure that the forms were filled in correctly and that there were uniform standards of recording of heart murmurs and other physical signs. After five years the conclusion was that there was no significant difference between the treatments as to final outcome. Nevertheless there were two advantages to cortisone over aspirin that were obvious to those who had the day to day care of the children. One was the rapid relief of painful pericarditis. The other was the rapid recovery of Wenckebach dysrhythmia and prolonged P-R interval on electrocardiography. This study ended in 1955. By then first-time admissions for rheumatic fever had almost disappeared, readmissions of children with established heart involvement were less frequent and the beds were filling instead with children and adults with chronic rheumatism.

With the change of clientele there followed a change in the scientific and clinical approach. Gadgets, many of them made on site, were invented to measure grip strength, finger joints swelling and ranges of joint motion. Perhaps some children now in their sixty's still have minute tattoo marks opposite their ankles, knees and greater trochanters which were made so as accurately to relocate a long arm goniometer for assessing changes in the range of movement of the knee. All observations were recorded on detailed charts.

The Rose Waaler test for rheumatoid factor was introduced in 1948 but even five years later there was still considerable debate as to what was and what was not rheumatoid arthritis in adults. In the USA Drs Walter Bauer, Granville (Red) Bennett and Marion Ropes took the view that they could see no histological difference between the synovial lesions of rheumatoid arthritis, psoriatic arthropathy and 'rheumatoid' (ankylosing) spondylitis and that these conditions could all be lumped together under rheumatoid arthritis. In continental Europe rheumatologists were diagnosing 'subacute rheumatism' and 'menopausal arthritis' as though they were differing entities. It was Bywater's achievement to sort this out. He redefined Type Jaccoud arthritis as a cause of benign ulnar deviation of the fingers in past sufferers from rheumatic fever and later, from systemic lupus. He introduced the concept of 'Adult onset Still's Disease' and like most European rheumatologists firmly differentiated ankylosing spondylitis and psoriatic arthropathy from rheumatoid arthritis on clinical grounds. He made important observations on the heart muscle and valve lesions of rheumatoid arthritis distinguishing these from those of rheumatic heart disease. For these and other important observations Bywaters was awarded the prestigious Gairdner Prize in 1962.

It is interesting that of the registrars in the 1947-1955 'rheumatic fever' period of Taplow, most became consultants in cardiology or general medicine. Only two stayed in rheumatology.

Barbara Ansell CBE, MD, FRCP, Hon FRCS, (Figure 7.2) qualified in Birmingham in 1946. She worked as House officer to Professor John McMichael at the Postgraduate Medical School in Hammersmith. An early contact with rheumatology occurred when she presented a case of scleroderma to Bywaters. She joined the staff at Taplow as Registrar in 1950 and apart from a spell as Senior Registrar at Hammersmith has worked there or at its successor hospitals ever since. From the first, Barbara always seemed a bit larger than life. Taplow had a quarter mile long corridor but her laugh was so strong that one could recognise it from the other end. Likewise her memory was extraordinary. She seemed to have instant recall of all the details of the children she had helped look after. She had the energy and perseverance to go with it. Bywaters relied more on his comprehensive files of all the manifestations of the children's diseases, their photographs, slides, histology, biopsies and X-rays. Between them they built up a unique body of knowledge, leading to many publications. One of these was a study of amyloidosis, a leading cause of death in Juvenile Chronic Arthritis (JCA). The prognosis for survival was much improved by chlorambucil treatment. Another was the observation that growth arrest caused by corticosteroid therapy could be minimised by alternate day dosage. Newer non-steroidal anti-inflammatory agents with a better therapeutic ratio replaced aspirin. The second line drugs used in adults, auranofin, hydroxychloroquine and penicillamine were found to be no better than placebos in JCA children. In 1959 Bywaters and Ansell published a new classification of JCA into pauci- (or oligo-) arthritis, poly-arthritis and systemic disease. The latter comprised the group dominated by fever, rash and enlargement of lymph nodes and spleen in which arthritis was sometimes a late or minor manifestation. This classification was based on mode of onset but was practical in that it helped with prognosis. The American Rheumatism Association and the World Health Organisation adopted it with minor modifications.

Fig 7.2. Dr Barbara Ansell

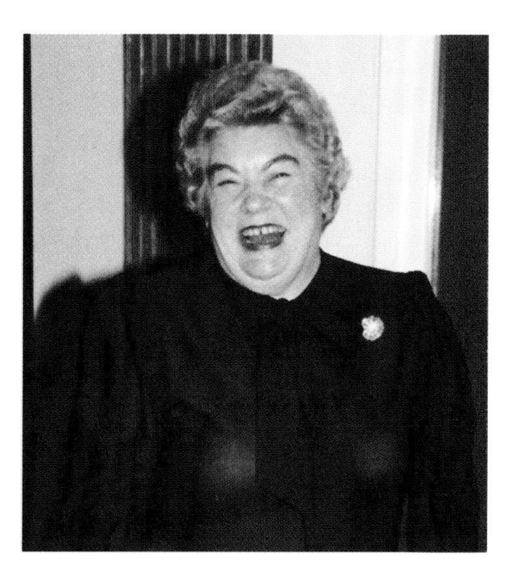

Until Bywaters retired in 1975 almost all the expertise in treating JCA had been developed at Taplow. The large number of affected children seen there enabled knowledge to be gained on all their

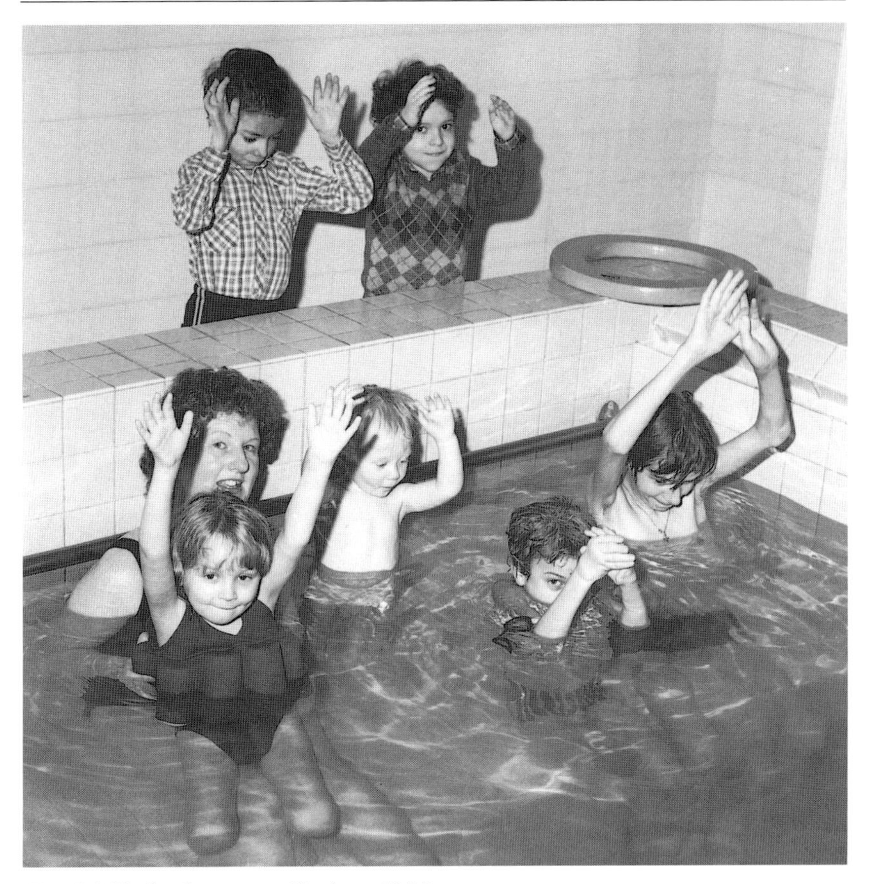

Fig 7.3 Hydrotherapy at Taplow, 1956

other problems. Many were successfully treated conservatively, using heat and anti-inflammatory drugs to reduce pain, with exercises and hydrotherapy to regain movement and muscle strength (Figure 7.3). At first there was only a ship's canvas bath but by 1956 a custom-made pool had been installed.

Nowhere more than in JCA did over-reliance on the theory of the curative powers of bed rest prove disastrous. Patients came to the Special Unit with a catalogue of bed-acquired deformities. The combination of flexion contractures of the knees with flexion-adduction of one hip and flexion abduction of the other hip was particularly unfavourable. (Figure 7.4)

Orthopaedic surgeon George Arden pioneered the use of hip and knee replacement arthroplasties in adolescents. There were some initial failures but later remarkable successes including children with all four joints replaced. Customised prostheses were developed. By 1975 he had replaced over 190 damaged hips (Ansell, 1998). Malcolm Swann followed him and is updating the book 'The Surgical Management of Juvenile Chronic Arthritis' published by Ansell and Arden (1975) to incorporate further technical improvements such as custom-made prostheses that have

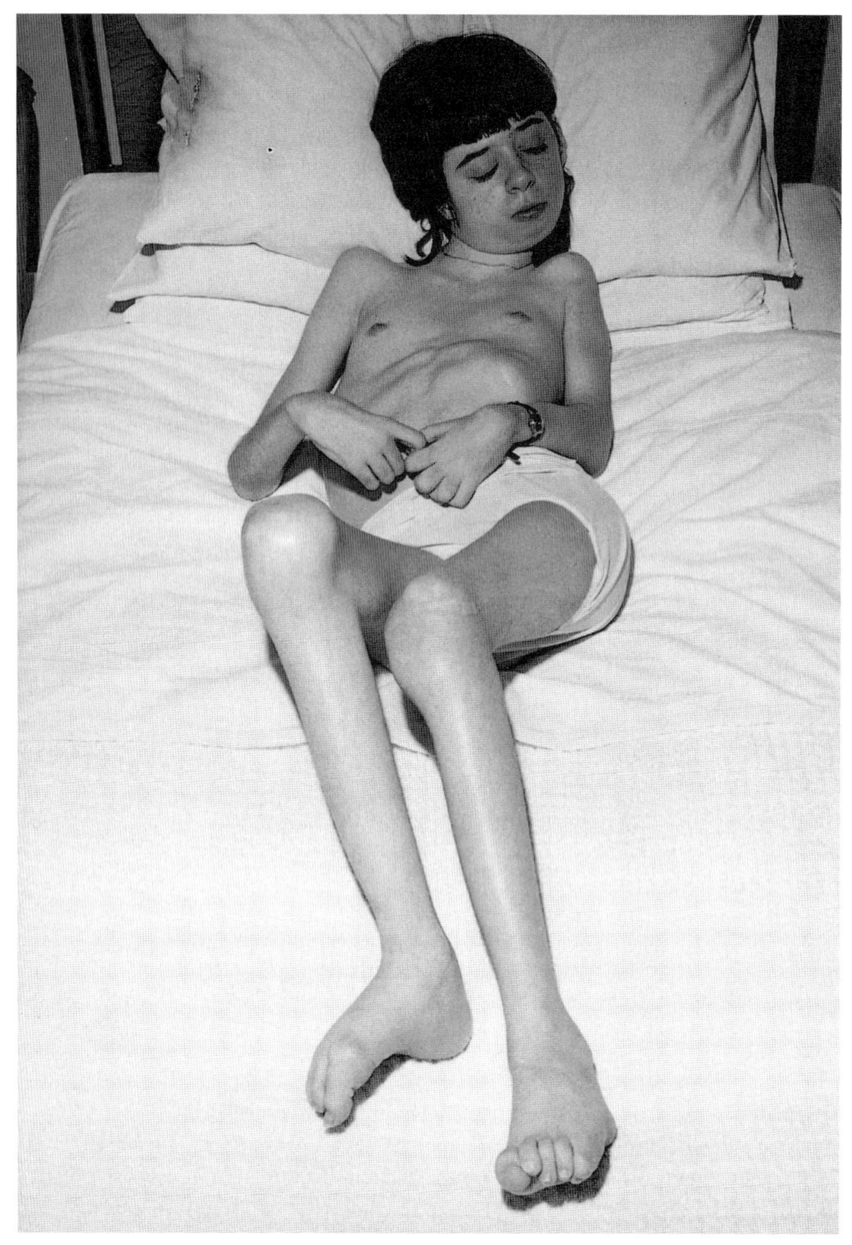

Fig 7.4. A teen-age girl with chronic arthritis showing multiple 'bed deformities'. In addition to the hip and knee contractures she shows generalised muscle wasting, dropped wrists, a stiff wry neck and contrasting deformities of the feet and toes

allowed hip replacement in small osteoporotic children. The youngest recipient was aged 9. Ankylosis or mutilans changes in the hands required the help of plastic surgeon Stewart Harrison.

Ophthalmologist Ken Smiley introduced prompt treatment with topical corticosteroids to abate inflammation and prevent synechiae in iridocyclitis. Jacek Kanski his successor emphasised that it was a medical emergency requiring even more vigorous treatment. Kanski also introduced a microsurgical method of removing cataracts in children and methods of treating secondary glaucoma. As a result blindness in children caused by 'Still's disease', once a substantial cause of acquired childhood blindness, became rare. Dental help was sometimes needed for children whose lower jaws had failed to grow or whose temperomandibular joints had fused. Children with stiffened necks presented enormous problems to anaesthetists.

Much credit must also go to the laboratory scientists. Dr (later Prof.) John Holborow studied the haemolytic streptococci, but as rheumatic fever disappeared his research gaze moved to immunology. He shared with Dr Jim Friou of the USA the proof that the LE factor was a gamma-globulin. Dr LE Glynn was in charge of the Unit's specialised pathology services and provided ideas for research, including animal models of inflammatory and osteoarthritic joints. He was later to become part-time Director of the Kennedy Institute. Biochemist Dr John Scott, previously with Kellgren at Manchester, developed ways of separating proteoglycans. Important others in the research team are described in Ansell and co-authors' book about ht hopsital, (1997)

Not all early deformities of the limbs were the result of damage to joints. Some reflected the periosteal reaction over the epiphyseal line, often seen in the X-rays of JCA. When this ossified it had the effect of stapling the growth plate, which might cause inequality of leg length or distortion of the forearm and lower leg when one of the parallel bones ceased to grow and the other did not. Sometimes a short metatarsal or metacarpal, usually the fourth, could result (Figure 7.5).

Early in its life, funding of the Special Unit was taken over by the Medical Research Council, a blessing in that it removed divisive money worries from the hospital's administrators. The cost of a patient on the Unit was, because of the research commitment, greater than that in the 'general' part of the hospital. It also implied a time bomb, as it was the Council's policy to close its units when the Director retired. And Bywaters did retire in 1975 and the Unit as such was closed. With his retirement Ansell extended her role to help other regions set up paediatric rheumatology clinics while maintaining a National Centre for Juvenile Rheumatism at the Medical Research Council Clinical Research Centre at Northwick Park. The services for JCA became dispersed but from the point of view of the child's family, nearer to home.

History can debate the benefits and disadvantages of assembling children with rheumatic and connective tissue diseases in one centre. The benefits are easy to list. A specialised hospital school can educate the children to work with head not hands. There is accurate differentiation of the different forms of JCA and expert and *experienced* management of the complications, including eye problems, limb deformities, renal amyloid and heart involvement. Proper documentation can be expected for rarities such as haemophilia and leukaemia presenting with arthritis, or for scurvy, osteomalacia or trichinella infestation mimicking polymyositis. Such a centre can build up experience of childhood osteoporosis whether idiopathic or corticosteroid induced. Finally such a centre will have less difficulty in the accretion of sufficient

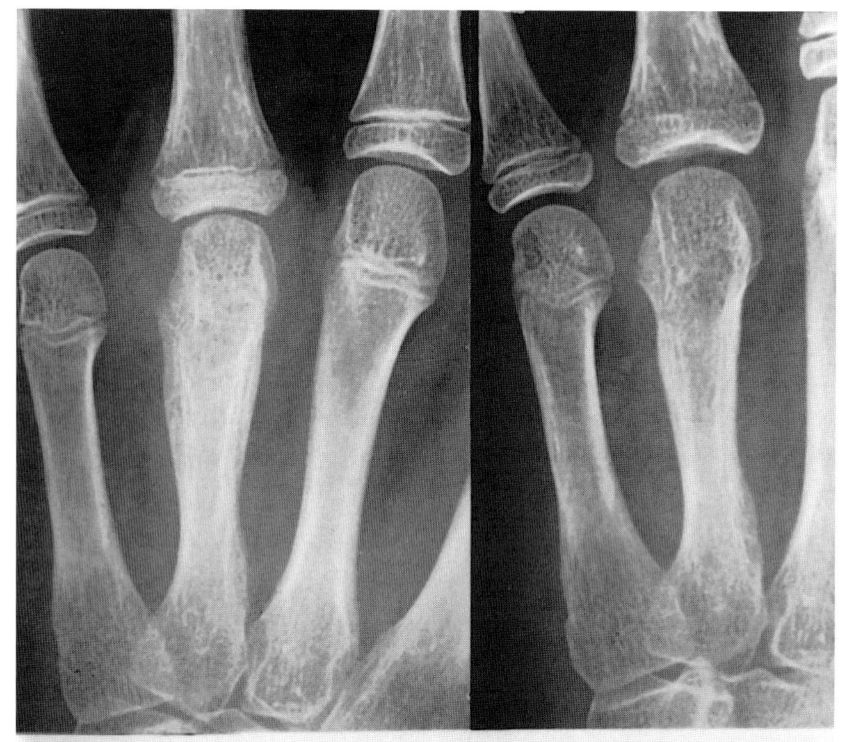

Fig 7.5. J.C., male, aged 13. Eighteen and twenty seven months from onset of Juvenile chronic arthritis showing subsiding periostitis of the fourth metacarpal with premature fusion of the epiphysis.

numbers of patients for clinical trials of new treatments or in the attraction of charitable funds to support research or to improve both the service offered and its public image.

But there are disadvantages, however imponderable. The main one is that the child may be distanced from its family for long periods with damage to family bonding, especially at the infant and toddler age, although Taplow had permission to pay parents who lived at a distance their travel costs to keep in touch.

And there can be blind spots. If a hospital sees only rheumatic diseases it may become blind to other conditions. A child was admitted with flitting limb pains and fever and diagnosed as 'possible rheumatic fever'. He next developed orchitis. The books were consulted. Yes, there was such a thing as rheumatic orchitis. It was not until he developed parotitis that the diagnosis of mumps was considered.

In 1988 Ansell retired although she continued her role as one of the early leaders of paediatric rheumatology through visits to other centres and countries. On a visit to a children's hospital in China, Prof. Paul Bacon noted that, despite the language barrier, she seemed to have instant rapport with the child patients.

The Hospital at Taplow did not long survive the loss of its Special Unit and the construction of a brand new general hospital for Slough at nearby Wexham Park. The buildings themselves became derelict. A commemorative history of the hospital and its special Unit was published (Ansell et al, 1997). The influence of Taplow is still apparent worldwide from the Fellows who trained there over the 30 years of its existence. A television programme in 1997 showed Dr Ansell walking round the ruined wards and reminiscing. The ghosts of children past seemed to be watching.

The baton of improving UK services for paediatric rheumatology passed largely to Prof. Pat Woo (Woo, 1997) at the Great Ormond Street Hospital for Sick Children and to Prof. Tauny Southwood at the Birmingham Children's Hospital.

Building on the Taplow legacy, moves were made in which Paediatric Rheumatology became a recognised speciality of medicine. Trainees could be taken on and two registrar posts approved and appointed. The British Paediatric Rheumatology Group grew from 10 to 100 members and has been allotted its own slot in the journal *Rheumatology*. By March 1997 there were a further 24 recognised services in England and Wales, three in Scotland and one in Northern Ireland.

Growth is expected in adolescent rheumatology services with the establishment of a clinic at the Middlesex Hospital, part of a centre for what used to be called ephebiatrics, but is now called adolescent medicine, at University College Hospital.

Ansell was asked how she saw the future for paediatric rheumatology when most major district hospitals could provide a service? Would the two main tertiary referral and academic centres in London and Birmingham find themselves without work? The answer was that adolescents have special needs that are still poorly catered for, often falling between paediatric and adult services. There were other problems to diversify into such as sports medicine in adolescents; sorting out the benign aches and pains of childhood from the serious rheumatic diseases; and work on the chronic fatigue syndrome in young people.

A crippled child in the family can be a divisive disaster or a unifying focus. Today medicine recognises the importance of the family in the total care concept and the stresses within the family that must be considered. The Children's Chronic Arthritis Association has taken on this role of family support. Annual holidays are arranged for the families, including the normal brothers and sisters. One hundred families have joined up with the Lady Hoare Trust for physically disabled children.

The European League against Rheumatism altered the constitution of the International and European Leagues so as to permit the setting up of Standing Committees to further the League's aims between congresses. One was the European Standing Committee on Paediatric Rheumatology, set up in 1979. The sub-varieties of JCA were not common and this move to European collaboration enabled larger studies to be made of the clinical manifestations, outcome and results of treatments with more statistical power. From this basis international co-operation became more systematised, with large conferences and the establishment of the Paediatrica Rheumatalogica International Trials Organisation (PRINTO), founded by Prof. A Martini (Italy), Prof. P Woo (UK) and Prof. M Prieur (France).

Chapter 8.
Surgical Rheumatology

The disappearance after the war of poliomyelitis, of rickets and of tuberculous and septic arthritis left many small orthopaedic hospitals without enough patients. William Waugh (1993) in his history of the British Orthopaedic Association noted that after the Festival of Britain in 1951 country orthopaedic surgeons found themselves out of work, although old habits died hard and many still insisted on weeks of bed rest after meniscectomy or hallux valgus operations. Some surgeons diversified into management of fractures, previously the domain of general surgeons and, following the pioneer work of Bradford and Spurling (1927) in the USA (Figure 8.1), undertook spinal surgery for back pain and sciatica caused by prolapsed intervertebral discs. Orthopaedics thus came to be the department of the hospital to which General Practitioners would send their patient with back, neck, foot and shoulder problems. For these complaints, and also for complaints of hip pain, orthopaedic surgeons *were* the rheumatologists. Even by 1960, relatively few hospitals had a rheumatologist on the staff and when one was appointed it was often the signal for setting up a combined medical and surgical approach to rheumatoid arthritis, particularly for sufferers whose disease had left them disabled and deformed through poor management.

Gout had been preventable since the introduction of probenecid and later allopurinol in the 1950s and '60s. Not many will recall that up to 1970 surgery was needed for the removal of large tophi (Figures 8.2) Thirty grams or more of sodium biurate could be removed in this way, thus reducing the time taken to clear the accumulations through the kidneys.

Fig 8.1. From p.46 of Bradford and Spurling (1941)

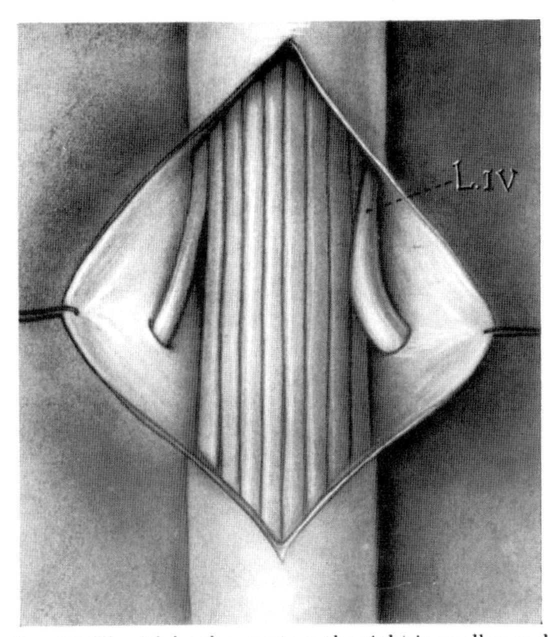

FIG. 20. The 4th lumbar root on the right is swollen and projects from its foramen in an abnormal manner. This may be the only evidence of root compression laterally in the intervertebral foramen.

Waugh recounted how for many years the British Orthopaedic Association tried to defend itself against splinter groups such as societies for research into hand surgery, paediatric orthopaedics, sports medicine, spinal manipulation, and podiatry. It was not until 1982 that these specialist societies were allowed to be affiliate to the Association and not until 1988 that the Rheumatoid Arthritis Surgical Society was affiliated. This was the only mention of rheumatology in his book, yet the surgery of arthritic joints had for thirty years been increasingly contributing to the orthopaedic surgeon's workload. (Conversely Kersley and Glyn's 'A Concise History of Rheumatology and Rehabilitation' made no mention of the extensive co-operation with orthopaedics in this period). The statistics issued by the Unit for Epidemiological Research of the Arthritis and Rheumatism Council, however, clearly showed the degree to which the public provision of rheumatological services depended on both specialities.

Mechanical problems of damaged joints demanded mechanical solutions. The Centre for Rheumatic Diseases in Glasgow published a contemporary cost/benefit analysis of

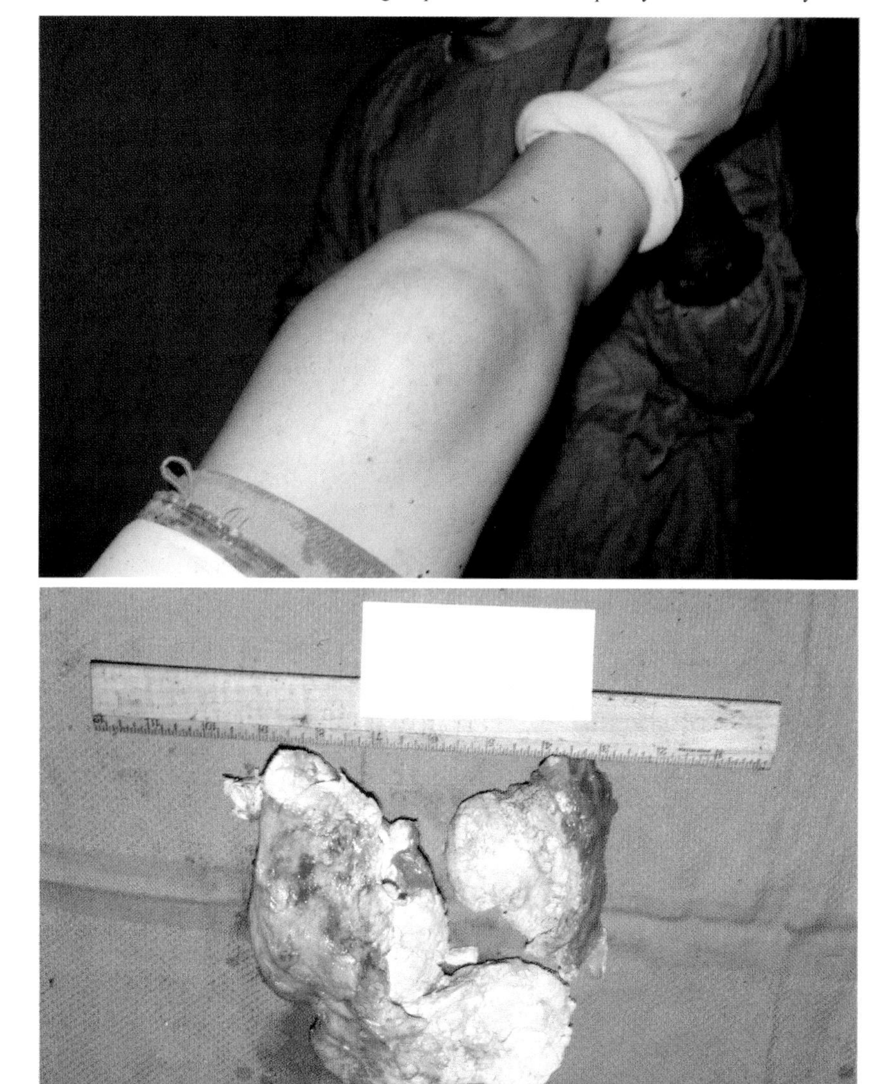

Fig 8.2. (a) A large tophus in the supra-patellar pouch which interfered with extension of the knee. (b) The deposit after removal.

treatment in rheumatoid arthritis that showed that in general the costs resulted from medical investigations and treatments. The economic benefits were predominantly surgical.

Of the surgical procedures the most beneficial has been the development of the total hip replacement arthroplasty. The late John Charnley is said to have wanted to set up a research unit for hip disease in the Manchester Royal Infirmary in the early 1950's when he was on the staff there but was not allowed to do so. So he offered to set it up in Wigan, at the Wrightington Hospital, an ex-tuberculosis hospital, where he was welcomed with open arms. His was not the first attempt to devise a total hip replacement. The key to his success was his use of cement to join metal to bone and the use of high molecular weight polyethylene in the acetabular socket. McKee, Ring and others had attempted to reproduce the size and shape of the femoral head and acetabulum and to fix their prostheses mechanically. Charnley saw that if one could reduce the diameter of the femoral head prosthesis and line the prosthetic acetabulum with a self-lubricating plastic there would be less friction and less wear (figure 8.4). Newman (1971) recounted the history of the development of hip prostheses. Total hip replacement was particularly suited to the older patient with osteoarthritis or rheumatoid arthritis. In younger, more vigorous subjects there was an up to 45% failure rate after 20 years. The procedure was adapted for disabling hip disease caused by ankylosing spondylitis, juvenile chronic arthritis and osteonecrosis. It was the treatment of choice for older osteoporotic patients with fractured neck of femur following the pioneering collaboration of RE Irving and M Devas (1967) at the orthogeriatric unit in Hastings, as it permitted rapid post-operative mobilisation. The incidence of fractured hip was increasing alarmingly, only partly explained by the increasing age of the population.

The success of the operation had created its own demand. With so many needing it and despite the obvious cost advantage of having patients pain-free and independent, long waiting lists built up in some areas, with pressure, almost scandalous, to transfer to the private sector. Shortage of staff, lack of dedicated ultra-clean operating theatre time and inefficient management of waiting lists were some of the reasons for the National Health Service's inability to cope. The standard of bacteriological hygiene that was required for joint replacement arthroplasty was very high. Few small private hospitals with only one operating theatre for both 'clean' and infected patients could meet that standard. The constraints that limited the number of NHS hip operations also limited the numbers of knee prostheses and to a lesser extent other operations such as osteotomies.

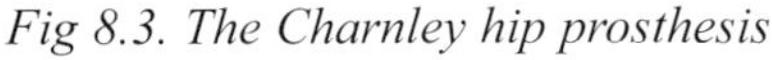
Fig 8.3. The Charnley hip prosthesis

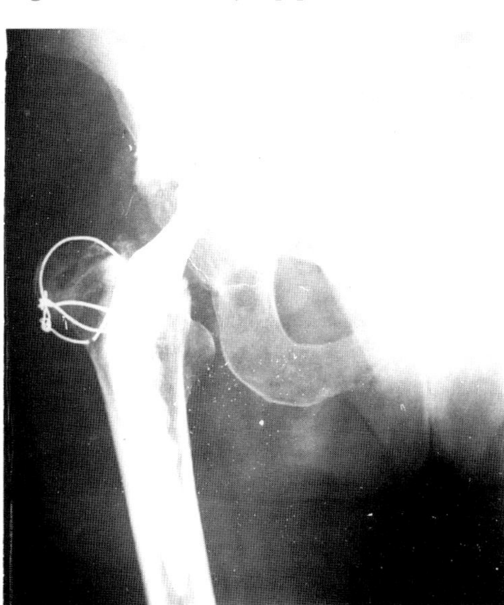

One of the earlier operations for rheumatoid arthritis was synovectomy, still occasionally required in the knee when the rheumatoid synovium is grossly hypertrophied. McCarty in the United States had described intra-articular injection of the corticosteroid triamcinalone hexacetonide in rheumatoid arthritis as a 'medical synovectomy'. Partly because of this and because of better medical measures to control the underlying disease both surgical synovectomy and intra-articular injections of radioactive synovial cauterising agents such as ^{90}Yttrium became rarely used.

Prostheses that have proved to reduce pain and improve function have been devised for all the larger limb joints.

Stabilisation of the neck was life saving when destruction of the joints at the top of the neck threatened to damage the spinal cord. Another salvage operation was the triple arthrodesis for ankle and hind foot joint destruction. In the hands, broken, frayed or displaced tendons could be repaired or replaced in their normal positions of function. Removal of the lower end of the ulna when it had undergone dorsal subluxation could restore wrist function. Excision osteotomies of the metatarsal heads could restore pain free walking to arthritic feet (Fig. 5.1). Knock-knee and bow-legged deformities could be corrected by wedge osteotomies or by hemi-arthroplasties, reviewed by Oliver (1997).

Metal or silicone prostheses were also designed for the wrists, fingers, thumb-base and first metatarsophalangeal joints. They have, on the whole, been less successful than the large joint replacements. Often the primary mechanical cause of impaired hand function was displacement, adhesion or rupture of tendons and unless those problems were solved a simple prosthesis would be likely to fail .

Patients with late Ankylosing Spondylitis ossified the discs and joints in their spines. If this happened in a patient who had retained an upright, almost military, posture the result in terms of function was reasonable, but too often such patients ossified in the position they were in when sitting. This was doubly unfavourable as the weight of the skull made the stiffened spine slowly remodel into greater and greater degrees of flexion until the unfortunate sufferer lost upward gaze when standing, and had to sit and tilt back to eat, to drink from a cup or to watch television. In very severe disease there was a danger of suffocation as the neck and head flexed to the point where the windpipe was compressed. For them spinal osteotomies have been successfully attempted at neck, thoracic and lumbar spinal levels, depending on where most of the kyphosis occurred.

Patients with chronic arthritis often had more than one joint requiring surgery. The decision then had to be made as to priority. In the lower limbs all those joints which made walking impossible needed to be tackled together or within a short time of each other otherwise rehabilitation was impossible. In the upper limbs a less radical approach was possible. In the past orthopaedic surgeons did not specialise in the surgery of any one joint. By 1998 in most modern hospitals there was sub-specialisation, surgeons operating on upper or lower limbs, but not both, and there were specialist hand surgeons and back surgeons. But close co-operation with rheumatologist colleagues helped ensure that medical complications would have less chance to spoil the surgeon's result.

Chapter 9
Charities:The Fourth Estate of Rheumatology

Dr Stephen Lock, when Editor of the British Medical Journal, used the phrase 'Fourth Estate of Medicine' to describe the 2000 or more non-governmental organisations, charities and self-help groups that worked for the interests of the sick and disabled.

Charitable giving throughout the latter half of the 20th century supported much of United Kingdom medical research and welfare. It benefited from the historical and non-political hierarchy of royalty, nobility and gentry who accorded their patronage and allowed their names to appear on the letterheads as Patrons or Presidents. It ensured stability and contrasted with charities in republican countries that looked to prominent politicians and industrialists for respectability and support and could find their fortunes change with the political and economic weather.

Charities had a social function for those who gave. A small village in one year might hold a dozen coffee mornings where people attended who might not otherwise meet each other. The local pub would have a 'Blind Night' and there would be amateur theatricals, concerts and public openings of private gardens in aid of a charity. The money raised was freely given and no government dared tax it.

The fund-raising charities that served people with rheumatic diseases fell into four groups. Broadly targeted organisations included the British Red Cross, Radar, the Lady Hoare Trust and the Disabled Living Foundation that supplied help and advice to adults or children with a wide range of physical disabilities. The Arthritis Research Campaign and the Oliver Bird Fund of the Nuffield Foundation were large charities aimed at rheumatology research and education. Next came the larger welfare organisations Arthritis Care, (previously called the British Rheumatism Association), and (in the past) the Horder Homes. Finally there was a host of smaller charities aimed at specific diseases such as Ankylosing Spondylitis or Osteogenesis Imperfecta.

Research organisations.

The Arthritis Research Campaign (ARC)

The Arthritis Research Campaign was started in 1928 as the 'National Campaign against Rheumatism' sponsored by Drs Lord Horder and Sir William Willcox. Dr Will Copeman who figured later would have been only three years qualified in medicine at the time. It was wound up in 1931 as a result of the prevailing economic depression but revived in 1935 with the recovery. In 1936 it was renamed 'The Empire Rheumatism Council' and known as the ERC until the word empire became inappropriate as the British colonies and dominions achieved independence and set up their own organisations. In 1962 the name was changed to the Arthritis and Rheumatism Council for Research, the 'for Research' tag distinguishing it from the British Rheumatism Association which was for welfare. The name changed again in 1997 to 'Arthritis Research Campaign' in the interests of orthology because the word

10 And may change again as rheumatology becomes increasingly concerned with soft tissue rheumatism, painful conditions of the back and diseases of bone not primarily related to arthritis.

'rheumatism' had lost meaning[10]. (Hench once defined rheumatism as 'any pain within a mile of a joint'). The new name retains the abbreviation ARC by which the Council was previously known.

The ARC immediately after World War 2 was a weak organisation. Its aims included treatment as well as research. In 1951 it became a public limited company and dropped the word treatment to distinguish it from other charities concerned with welfare. Both Horder, who was the King's physician, and Copeman, who followed him as Chairman of the ARC in 1953, were Harley Street consultants of renown. Fund raising for the ARC in the early days depended largely on persuading their rich and influential patients and their contacts to give large sums of money. The ARC had no formal membership of ordinary citizens who would pay a small annual subscription to belong to the organisation. Under Copeman's chairmanship the ARC continued to aim its fundraising mainly at big money donors. Copeman had married Helen Bourne, of the London retailers 'Bourne and Hollingsworth' family and through them had recruited help and funding from other Oxford Street storeowners, John Spedan Lewis and Gordon Selfridge. This was the system Copeman knew and trusted. But as firms owned by private families became public limited liability companies the money became harder to get. It was necessary instead to approach industrialists and hard headed directors, so in 1949, 1954 and 1959 the ARC set up campaigns to raise money from industry and commerce. These were only partly successful, falling short of their targets. The donations to the ARC, mainly from large sum givers, fell from £15,652 in 1938 to £7,315 in 1939 and by the end of the war were down to £2,842. Between November and December 1948 the ARC finances were in deficit. Sir Stanley Davidson, Professor of Medicine at Edinburgh and the King's Physician in Scotland, was Chairman of the ARC's Scientific Advisory Committee. He went so far as to suggest that the ARC should be wound up. But the ARC was soon back in credit. The country became more prosperous and, despite growing competition from rheumatism welfare organisations, income gradually rose. Even so it would be a long time before the ARC could match the funds available to The Nuffield Foundation.

The discovery of cortisone in 1948 had considerably increased the public interest in rheumatic diseases but rival organisations also benefited. "Such was the disparity in income that The Nuffield Foundation allocated more money to cortisone research in its Manchester Unit, (£5,600 for additional staff) than the ARC spent on all research in 1949-50." (Cantor).

Nevertheless by the end of the 1950s the ARC's annual income quadrupled to £68,000, enabling it to expand its research. At that time donations constituted 73% or more of the ARC's income and only a small part from legacies. These proportions were to change radically in later years.

After the war Victor Howell became the Executive Secretary of the ARC but by 1955 was dying of cancer. Michael Andrews succeeded him the following year. Andrews brought a less elitist philosophy into fundraising. Instead of pursuing the rich patients of the Harley Street doctors and the captains of industry and commerce he tried a broader approach. The 1959 appeal that had already been planned went ahead but fell £100,000 pounds short of its target of £250,000. The relative success of the two welfare organisations, the British Rheumatism Association and the Horder Centres, which during the 1950's had established local branches, was not lost on Andrews. Andrews set about developing the ARC's own regional organisation and aiming appeals more at the ordinary man and woman.

In 1961 the ARC established its first regional organisations in the Northwest, Southeast, Yorkshire, Scotland and Wales regions and other regional organisations followed in the West Midlands (1964), North London and Home Counties (1966), Southwest (1967), Borders (1969), Southern Counties (1970) and East Anglia (1970). Each paid Regional Secretary had to publicise the ARC and set up local committees and branches. A seam of energy and good will, previously un-mined, was exposed. New ways to raise money were devised. Thus in 1974 a tiny group of ARC supporters in the village of St. Keverne in Cornwall invented the ARC Knit-in. Their women members all had bits of leftover knitting wool in their workboxes. They decided to knit these into nine inch squares and then sew them together to make colourful blankets or rugs which could be sold. This idea cost nothing but the voluntary labour. It was taken up all over the country and made a useful contribution to the ARC's income.

The first local branch of ARC was formed in Cheshire in 1961 and when Andrews retired in 1983 there were over 900 branches, increasing to over 1000 in 1997. A magazine, entitled 'ARC', was founded by Andrews and the information officer Patrick Lacey. It was of considerable help in recruiting new branches. By 1970 Dora

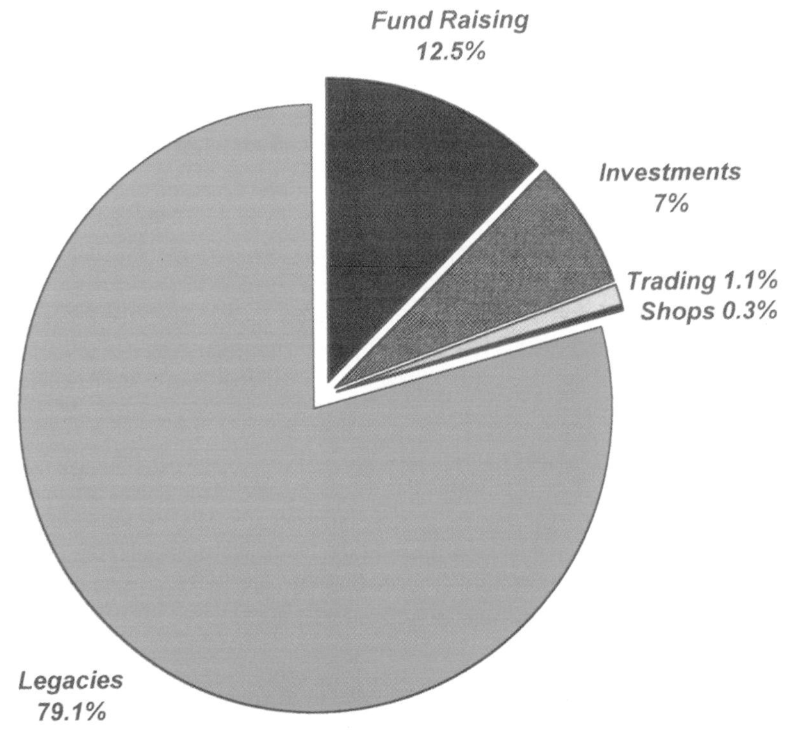

Bolitho, the Regional Secretary for the Southwest, had formed 60 branches, most of them in her native Cornwall, outstripping the efforts of the other regional secretaries.

The branches did not always toe the line of national policy. In 1971 the Consett branch assisted the rheumatoid arthritis sufferer Lila Dodds to buy an electrically driven wheel chair, a job which should have fallen to the British Rheumatism Association according to the informal demarcation agreement whereby the ARC supported research and the Association supported welfare. At a later date Dr Barbara Ansell was to sit on governing committees of both organisations and could help ensure co-ordination of strategy.

The continuing success of smaller scale fundraising by large numbers of branches contrasted with the relative failures of named, centrally run campaigns but it could bring its own problems. Localism could become a hindrance to the spirit of national unity that had endured during and immediately after the war. In the provincial cities people were worried about their own problems as industry faced expensive readjustment and foreign competition. In a co-operative appeal in Birmingham the ARC found that the local chairman refused to let any money jointly raised pass through the books of the ARC. To counter such localism the ARC set up a protected West Midlands fund and also a Scottish fund to be spent only on local projects. But those who wished to draw on the funds still had to go before the ARC's Research Subcommittee for approval.

The system of regional organisers and local branches did much to harness and tame localism. One further advantage soon became very apparent. People made money in the cities but retired to the country. There they had time and energy to become involved in local ARC activities and there they made their wills. Residuary estates were particularly helpful benefactions. A will made five years before death might give specified sums and chattels to relatives, but the value of a residuary estate could double in five years because of inflation and the rise in house prices.

Other sources of income that were set up in the 1970s and '80s were a trading company that sold Christmas Cards and gifts, and charity shops run by volunteers. A glance at its annual accounts would suggest that neither the trading company nor the charity shops were money-spinners for the ARC; they raised only marginally more than they cost to run. But by involving local people in this way the ARC built up local loyalties and when these supporters made their wills they remembered the ARC.

By 1983 Andrews as Executive Secretary had seen the ARC's gross annual income rise to over £5m and it was to rise to over £21m under the care of his successor, Jim Norton. The steady increase allowed the ARC to spend more on rheumatism research and education than did the Nuffield Foundation. The ability to fund long term commitments was assured. By 1997 just under 80% of the ARC's £17,268,000 spendable income came from legacies (Fig. 9.1).

11 Numbers in brackets refer to the number of committee members and others entitled to attend in 1998.

Spending the money, the committee structure

If the ARC were to improve the lot of rheumatic disease sufferers it needed to address research into those diseases and the education of those who would diagnose and treat them. Accordingly in the early 1950s the Research Advisory Committee became the Scientific Co-ordinating Committee (22)[11] that had two sub committees, the Research Sub committee (17) and the Education Sub committee (19). At a later date it added two more, the Committee for Academic Development (10) and the Fellowship Committee (variable).

There was at first a hierarchical structure. Younger consultants invited to the Education Subcommittee would have to work their passage by contributing to the *Reports on Rheumatic Diseases* which dealt with practical problems and which were circulated free of charge to general practitioners. The *Reports* were important in showing practitioners that rheumatology was not just another name for physical medicine or spa treatment. This committee had by 1988 developed Working Groups on Undergraduate Education, Postgraduate Education, Allied Health Professionals, Educational Grants to Individuals, Educational grants to Institutions, and one on Publications. It was a spending committee but was never allowed to stray into major expenditure. In 1998 it spent less than 1% of total disbursements.

Some of those who had served on the Education Committee might proceed to the Research Committee. There they would join a team of scientists representing a variety of disciplines that were considered relevant to rheumatology research. In the early days of the ARC this was where most of the available funds were allocated. By 1998 this committee accounted for 36% of all research expenditure and the Fellowships Committee for 14%. The Scientific Co-ordinating Committee recommended core grants to the Kennedy Institute (18%) and the Epidemiology Research Unit (8.5%)

Since 1953 the ARC pursued a policy, whenever it had the money, of establishing Professorial Chairs of Rheumatology in suitable universities. The first Chair had been accorded in 1953 to JH Kellgren at Manchester and the second in 1957 to EGL Bywaters in Hammersmith. Chairs were generally endowed for ten years. By 1998 there were seven fully and one partly endowed ARC Chairs. There were also 27 Senior Lecturerships that the ARC financed, usually for five years, before they were taken over by the universities. There were only six medical schools where there had been no ARC-supported senior academic posts. The large expenditure on academic posts contrasted with the relatively low funding of education as judged by the work of the Education Committee. Dr Colin Barnes when Chairman of the ARC explained that the word academic was interpreted as research but that the presence of an academic Department of Rheumatology in a medical school would be expected also to improve the standard of undergraduate education.

Rheumatology research, ad hoc or directed?

Most of the scientific research supported by the Research Committee over the years has been ad hoc. The Committee was reactive, it could only consider the proposals put to it. It could not take a proactive stance and plan or direct research. In the early 1970s when Dr Philip Wood was working on the distribution of named rheumatic diseases in the UK, the ARC used his statistics for fund raising, claiming that 1 in 4 of the adult members of the public suffered from a rheumatic condition. On analysis most were complaints of back pain. At the time the ARC was funding little directly related to back pain. This led to an attempt to direct research into three areas of perceived need, identified as the development of a knee prosthesis as good as the hip prostheses, the discovery or exclusion of a microbial cause for rheumatoid arthritis, and research into the causes and treatment of back pain. These were advertised but proposals still required the ARC's Research Committee's approval. There was a small surge in the number of back pain related projects submitted few of which were considered to have scientific merit when compared, for example, to proposals dealing with the immunology of rheumatoid arthritis. There were no new ideas for detecting infection in rheumatoid arthritis and it was pointed out that promising work on a prosthesis for the knee was already being funded elsewhere.

Back pain had long been the province of orthopaedic surgeons and heterodox healers, the latter claiming success for their various methods but unaware of the high natural recovery rate. There were few controlled trials of treatments for back pain. Back pain science was far less mature than arthritis science and stood little chance of obtaining ARC Research Committee approval. The solution seemed to be to establish a scientific forum on back pain outside the ARC ambit. In 1973 the interdisciplinary Society for Back Pain Research was set up. The Society was open to all who were interested in the problem. The only condition was that papers and studies should be communicated to the Society for criticism and review. With time standards of research improved.

Another reason for considering directed research was dissatisfaction with the practical results of that which had been supported. There had by the 1970s been three major advances in rheumatology. These were the cure of gout, the disappearance of rheumatic fever and rheumatic heart disease, and Charnley's work on the low friction hip arthroplasty. One could ask the question, how much had ARC-funded research contributed to these advances? The answer was not a lot. The ARC had refused a grant to Charnley in the early stages of his work.

Time was when the ARC Research Committee interviewed all applicants for funding. The applicant had the chance to clarify points raised in discussion and the Committee could judge the scientist as well as the science. With the increasing workload this became too time consuming and it was decided to consider only written submissions. Efforts were made to make the selection process as objective as possible. Applications were sent to external assessors and application forms were standardised. Projects were scored according to a set protocol. The effect was often to favour larger institutions with 'professional' expertise in writing applications for research funding. A well-written application went a long way towards convincing a committee that a project was worth financing, even if not particularly original.

It was recognised that the system could tend to select the mediocre and miss the new ideas because the applicant was impatient of following the prescribed paths when applying. The work of Professor Graham Hughes was a case in point. He had a series of applications to ARC turned down because they were badly presented. Yet his research work was innovative and his scientific papers on the anticardiolipin antibody in systemic lupus were published in high quality peer-reviewed scientific journals. Meanwhile the Research Committee's paperwork expanded exponentially and what could in the 1960s be dispatched in two hours in 1998 extended over two days. There was no easy solution.

Setting up Research Units.

If research could not be directed it was at least possible to set up research units with defined areas in which to work. In 1956 the Mobile Field Unit at Manchester had been established. It was partly supported with ARC money to investigate the spinal and joint morbidity of miners in the Lancashire coalfields, as mentioned in Chapter 2, and to make epidemiological surveys of rheumatic diseases in other populations. In 1959 the ARC established an industrial research unit in Edinburgh to investigate rheumatic complaints in industries and relate these to working conditions and days lost from work. (There was an ulterior motive in this, the ARC had set up a special campaign aimed at getting industrialists to support its work and it was necessary to show that it was doing something to reduce the toll of working days lost to industry because of occupational hazards). In 1961 it endowed for ten years a Unit for Drug Action at King's College Hospital under the direction of Dr MJH Smith. This explored the intermediary metabolism of salicylates and related anti-rheumatic drugs and took part in the ARC-sponsored International Symposium on Salicylates in 1962.

In 1967 Dr PHN Wood took over the Manchester Mobile Field Unit and renamed it the ARC Unit for Epidemiological Research. He improved the quality and computer handling of data collection and updated the rubrics related to rheumatic complaints in the International Classification of Diseases (9th and 10th editions). He used this to count named complaints and relate them to geographical areas and occupations. He extended the concept of epidemiology from counting diseases in populations to counting and analysing the community resources available to cope with them. This led him into studying the numbers and distribution of orthopaedic surgeons, 'physicians with an interest', rheumatologists and physical medicine specialists. His lists of the various categories of professionals were often more accurate than those of the Department of Health. He looked at training in rheumatology, the roles of 'Professions Allied to Medicine' and the contributions of heterodox healers. As with the earlier work of the Edinburgh Industrial Research Unit the findings had important public relations effects on the ARC's fundraising. If Cornwall or Cumberland were relatively deprived of resources for rheumatism sufferers when compared with London or Liverpool, the ARC Regional Secretaries had persuasive arguments for increasing local fund raising. Moreover appeals to the pride of members of local hospital authorities could stimulate them to remedy defects.

He was later to become involved in definitions of disability in connection with the World Heath Organisation. In Australia he had listened to the invited speaker at a conference on disability. The speaker had a severe impairment. He had been born without arms but he had adapted to this in such a way that he had relatively little disability. He gave his talk and skilfully turned the pages of his notes with his toes.

Wood says this set him thinking about the definitions of handicap and disability, relevant at that time because of the Amelia Harris survey of disability in the population in relation to the Chronic Sick and Disabled legislation.

For the World Health Organisation, Wood prepared the International Classification of Impairment, Disability and Handicap. The differences were defined because they were often used loosely and as though they were interchangeable. *Impairment* was the loss of a part or a function, such as loss of hearing, or loss of an arm. *Disability* described the functions or activities that the subject was unable to perform, and *Handicap* was the disadvantage imposed on the subject when compared to those without the impairment. This underpinned the analysis of disabilities in relation to lifestyle and jobs. A man born without hands who could use his feet and toes with the skill and precision that is taken for granted in the hands would have many handicaps but one of them was not the ability to earn a living as a speaker or writer.

Wood became in effect the ARC's contact man with the government, submitting a report on behalf of the ARC for the Merrison Commission on the Future of the National Health Service and taking a leading part in the government's Back Pain Working Party. The Working Party analysed all the literature on the treatment of back pain. The vast majority of papers considered had to be rejected as anecdotal and uncontrolled. The small number where scientific methods of evaluation were evident became even smaller when their perceived relevance to the back pain problem was taken into account.

Prof. Wood qualified from St Bartholomew's Medical School in 1955. He had entered the medical profession relatively late having spent National Service in the army as a hygiene inspector. At Kyoto in the Congress of the International League Against Rheumatism he sat with a typewriter and, despite interruptions and noise all round, typed out new and word-perfect Constitutions for the European and International Leagues. This included the provisions for Standing Committees that were to continue the work of the Leagues between congresses. It also imposed limited terms of office on the members of the governing committees of the Leagues, getting rid of sinecures.

In his role of epidemiologist concerned with the resources available for rheumatism sufferers, Wood took an interest in the split between rheumatology and physical medicine. That split was more organisational than founded in professional practice. In 1964 a private meeting of younger consultants had taken place to discuss the possibilities of a merger. It was already apparent that there was a 70% dual membership of the Heberden Society and the British Society for Physical Medicine. ARC records showed that Copeman got to hear about the meeting and took steps to make sure the 'urge to merge' got no further at that time. Ordinary members of the societies might see no problem but the leaderships of the two societies valued the offices they held and had an interest in keeping them apart. It took some years of patient persuasion by Wood and others before the merger took place and the situation was rationalised.

Wood retired in 1988 and was succeeded by Professor Alan Silman.

Other Research Units were funded that were not targeted at any particular aspect of the fight against the rheumatic diseases. The ARC established the first electron microscopy Unit at St Thomas' Hospital. In 1964 the ARC contributed to the establishment of a Research Institute of Rheumatology at the Arthur Stanley institute of the Middlesex Hospital. In 1965 the ARC established a Research Department of Rheumatology at the Royal London Hospital Medical School and in 1976 built a Bone and Joint Research laboratory there. There were at the time three productive young consultants, Dr Harry Currey, (rheumatologist, from South Africa and Hammersmith Hospital), Dr Barry Vernon Roberts, pathologist and Mr Michael Freeman, an active and resourceful orthopaedic surgeon. All were co-operating as joint directors of the Bone and Joint Research Unit but had no common premises. But Vernon Roberts went to Australia and the building was used for a variety of purposes until the appointment of David Blake in 1983 as ARC Professor of Rheumatology with a mission to explore the role of reactive free radicals in arthritis. In 1982 the ARC gave substantial sums to help set up the Bath Institute of Rheumatic Diseases in association with Bath University and the Royal National Hospital for Rheumatic Diseases. ARC endowments of Professorial Chairs usually carried with them funds for Associated Lecturers and Research Assistants.

The ARC and the Kennedy Institute.

The Kennedy Institute was the largest research centre that the ARC helped to set up. In 1961 Mathilde and Terence Kennedy had given £500,000 to establish an Institute of Rheumatology and the ARC had guaranteed £200,000 over 5 years to run it. The offer was accepted by the Charing Cross Hospital, which was contemplating its move to the Fulham Palace Road. One floor of the new hospital was to be adopted as the Kennedy Institute. Shortage of funds caused the reduction in the number of floors from 22 to17 and this meant that the new Institute had to be built in Bute Street, behind the West London Hospital. The Institute was finally opened on the 5th of October 1966, five years after the money was offered.

Dr Dugald Gardner, who had worked with Duthie in Edinburgh and was previously a Lecturer in Pathology there was the first Director of the Institute. In his memoir printed in the 31st annual report of the Kennedy Institute he wrote:

The [opening] ceremony was held partly within the elegant ground floor vestibule of the Institute, partly in the covered grounds that lay around the pool and fountain. Dr WSC Copeman, Chairman of the Arthritis and Rheumatism Council for Research at that time, was Physician to Members of the Royal Household, and the Duke and Duchess of Gloucester had graciously agreed to perform the opening ceremony. There were present dignitaries from the worlds of medicine, science, politics and the arts. The London 'Times' carried a Supplement to mark the occasion. Lord Porritt, President of the ARC, sat in the front row. The Mayor of Hammersmith and representatives of firms of architects, companies associated with the building and suppliers of all kinds were happily present.'

The Institute was to have divisions of biochemistry, biology, clinical investigation, immunology, microbiology and experimental pathology. In addition it had a conference room, a library and workshop and offices. It was also to advance public and professional education about the rheumatic diseases. It had its own management committee and in 1969 was registered as a separate charity and a company limited by guarantee. Gardner estimated that its running costs would escalate in a few years to £150,000 pa or more. Finding that money became increasingly difficult. The Kennedy Institute accounted for about 4% of ARC expenditure in 1965, 33% in 1966 and to over 37% in 1970. Even so the work of the Institute might have had to be curtailed or the Institute itself wound up unless further funds could be found. Eventually the Executive Committee of ARC took over responsibility for the management of the Kennedy Institute and made it the theme of a major National appeal for £1m headed by Lord Kindersley.

The cost to the ARC of subsidising the Kennedy Institute upset some members of the Research Committee who regarded it as an expensive cuckoo in the nest. Their reservations were overcome as the Institute was increasingly seen as a success and a credit to the ARC.

Dugald Gardner was regarded by some of the staff of the Institute as not an easy man to get on with, hardly surprising perhaps when he was battling with the shortage of funds in the early days but at the same time building up the research programmes. At first he was assisted by an accountant, necessary because some Kennedy money had been spent on medical research before his arrival and before the Institute was opened. Later he was assisted with managerial tasks by a Mr McNeil as General Secretary when the Kennedy Institute became incorporated. Gardner was also head of the Division of Experimental Pathology and was an expert on the newer methods of microscopy. A notable paper he wrote was entitled 'Articular cartilage is not smooth', in which he drew attention to the tiny undulations of the surface of cartilage, trapping small amounts of synovial fluid during movement as a form of weeping lubrication. This provided an explanation for the extraordinarily low coefficient of friction in mammalian joints, better than any engineering joint other than roller bearings.

One of Gardner's first appointments as Director was Helen Muir who was at the time studying the biochemistry of atherosclerosis under difficult conditions in another hospital. Gardner took Muir to tea in a Lyons teashop over Hammersmith Station and offered her the job of Head of the Division of Biochemistry. She accepted at once. He asked her 'don't you want to know about the terms and conditions of the appointment?' The answer was no. She had private funds and a property in Yorkshire. She just wanted to be free to get on with her work in better surroundings. Within two days she and her assistant Roger Ewens had put their chromatography columns in a taxi and moved in. The appointment of Dr Joe Chayne as head of the Division of Biology was a different matter. He and Dr Lucille Bitenski, whom he later married, were working at the laboratories of the Royal College of Surgeons in Lincoln's Inn Fields. They too had been involved in research into heart disease. Joe was much more legalistic, wanted everything cut and dried beforehand and amongst his conditions for accepting was one that, as an orthodox Jew, he must be free to leave work before sundown on a Friday. He would compensate, he said, by coming in on Sundays. Gardner remembers, wryly, that he didn't come into work on Sundays, so 'He had the best of both worlds'. Chayne was an expert on microscopic biochemical analysis and used this to identify the metabolism of synovial surface lining cells so as to distinguish it from that of the underlying connective tissue. Later he was involved in the discovery of the role of Vitamin K in the production of osteocalcin, one of the non-structural proteins in bone and a marker for osteoporosis. Dr Dudley Dumonde, previously with Bywaters at Hammersmith, was appointed Head of the Division of Immunology. Dumonde had done early work in the emerging field of cytokines. Dr Tom Scott who was on the staff of the Kennedy Institute as part of his appointment in 1966 as Consultant Physician and Rheumatologist to the Charing Cross Hospital, became Deputy Director and Head of the Clinical Division.

After five years Gardner returned to Scotland to resume a preferred career in teaching. By that time the numbers of people employed in the Institute had risen from one to one hundred and over a hundred scientific papers and many reports had been written.

Dr Leonard Glynn, also a pathologist, was the next Director, part time. He was described as more easy-going. He was also Senior Pathologist at the Special Unit at for Juvenile Rheumatism at Taplow. Glynn was succeeded by an 'in-house' promotion of Dr Helen Muir as Director. Dumonde left at this point to take on a senior position in St Thomas' Hospital. Muir was a brilliant biochemist and was largely responsible for unravelling the structure of the glycosaminoglycans and showing that there was a protein core to the carbohydrate macromolecule. On her retirement she was succeeded by Professor R Maini, clinician and immunologist.

The premises in Bute Street became clinically 'orphaned' when the West London Hospital next door closed all but for maternity services. The Institute was later moved into the Sunley building in the grounds of the new Charing Cross Hospital. It was not until Maini's time in 1990 that medical students came to the Kennedy. With the Institute involved in treatment and clinical work it was having no, or at any rate less, difficulty in funding.

Had the Kennedy Institute fulfilled the aspirations of its founders? As an internationally famous rheumatism research centre, yes. As a leader and reference centre for the whole of the United Kingdom rheumatology the answer had to be no. It came on the scene too late for that. Other research centres had by then multiplied and established their own networks of co-operation and advice. Moreover there was no consistent policy for dispersing professional talent developed in the Institute. Unlike the Postgraduate Medical School, which was viewed as a training centre and where all but the most senior were on fixed term contracts, the Kennedy tended to hang on to its people. Thus when Helen Muir was offered a senior job in Sheffield University changes were made in order to keep her. Had she gone to Sheffield she would have been doing the same work at no cost to ARC, which could then have opened up another line of research.

ARC finance and investments,

Throughout its history a Finance and Investment Committee advised the ARC Executive Committee. It consisted of distinguished financial experts from the City of London. Lord Kindersley who was at one time the President of ARC and had been the Governor of the Bank of England may have helped select those experts. Kindersley was himself a rheumatism sufferer. After 1950 the ARC began to accumulate a financial reserve that with the rise of the stock market built up a substantial capital base. But there were hitches. On one occasion the Chairman of the Finance Committee was proud to announce that that he had transferred all the ARC's gilt-edged securities investments into equities. The very next day the stock market fell heavily! On another occasion, when the Committee was meeting in a cigarette smoke-filled room in the Royal College of Physicians, which had an anti-smoking policy, the suggestion was made that ARC should not invest in the tobacco industry. The response was that the Investment committee could not be tethered in any way and must be free to obtain the best return on the ARC's money. This was an untenable position for a health related organisation and when a member of the Church Commissioners' Investment Committee was consulted he was of the opinion that it was quite practical, and did not entail a financial sacrifice, to direct investments away from businesses considered unethical. By 1998 it was known from research in Norfolk that cigarette smoking was a positive risk factor for rheumatoid arthritis. The battle to stop smoking in the Royal College of Physicians building was eventually won.

The ARC and the Heberden Society

From the beginning there had been a somewhat incestuous relationship between ARC and the Heberden Society, the professional learned society for rheumatology. For a start there was much cross-membership of the governing bodies. Copeman was Chairman of the ARC and also Honorary Librarian of the Heberden Society and Dudley Hart was on the committees of ARC and was Honorary Treasurer of the Society. Unlike other members of the Heberden Executive they did not have limited terms of office and could attend all meetings year in and year out. The ARC under Copeman's Chairmanship made a regular grant in aid to the Society for its expenses. The two organisations shared the same headquarters. The Society's administration and secretarial work were carried out by the Executive Secretary of ARC until 1983 when the Heberden Society merged with the British Association of Rheumatology and Rehabilitation to become the British Society for Rheumatology. At that point the combined organisation set up its own independent secretariat. It also had its own Education Standing Committee that was finding a *modus vivendi* with the Education Committee of ARC.

Oliver Bird Fund of the Nuffield Foundation

In 1943 when Lord Nuffield had started the Nuffield Foundation with a donation of £1,000,000's worth of shares in Morris Motors £180,000 was earmarked for rheumatism research. In 1947 Captain Oliver Bird of 'Bird's Custard' fame gave £450,000 to the Nuffield Foundation 'for research into prevention and cure of rheumatism'. In 1947 Sir John Stopford was Vice Chancellor of Manchester University and also Chairman of the Nuffield Foundation. Under his Chairmanship the Foundation granted £10,000 annually for ten years to establish the 'University of Manchester Centre for Rheumatic Diseases'. Dr JH Kellgren was appointed in charge of the clinical section with consultant status in the Manchester Royal Infirmary, the Withington Hospital, and the Devonshire Royal Hospital at Buxton. In 1953 he was elected Professor after Stopford persuaded the ARC to endow a Chair. Professor SL Baker headed the pathology section, joined later by Dr John Ball.

Laboratory research work began on the premise that the inflammatory rheumatic diseases were disorders of connective tissue. Accordingly collagen, interstitial ground substance and fibrinoid were explored for their biochemistry and turnover. Collaboration with Professor Astbury of Leeds University showed that the collagen present in rheumatoid nodules was unaffected by cortisone treatment. Clinical studies and epidemiological surveys were begun. By 1952, the Nuffield Committee was sufficiently impressed by the Manchester unit to increase and extend the grant.

The University of Edinburgh Rheumatic Unit which had been established in 1947 under the leadership of Dr JJR Duthie was allocated a grant of £12,319 over five years by the Oliver Bird Fund in 1949 for the assessment of therapies in arthritis, including the effects of cortisone and adrenocorticotrophic hormone. There were other substantial grants. Grants for corticosteroid-related research went to Birkbeck College, Glasgow University and the Middlesex Hospital. By 1954 hopes that cortisone research would result in the cure of inflammatory rheumatism had faded. In pursuit of those hopes the Nuffield Foundation had given £70,000 to the Manchester Rheumatism Unit, £27,000 to Edinburgh, £10,000 to St Mary's, £8,000 to Sheffield, and £6,000 to Stoke Mandeville Hospital and smaller sums to Birkbeck College, Glasgow University and Middlesex Hospital.

Of long-term clinical significance was a grant in 1949 to support Dr Marcia Wilkinson's original work on the painful syndromes arising from cervical disc diseases. There was also a grant to Dr EGL Bywaters to continue a study of 250 patients with conventionally treated rheumatoid arthritis, started in 1939. A grant made to Cambridge for a survey of the prevalence of rheumatic complaints in a rural population discovered a number of persons who had severe rheumatoid arthritis yet who had never been to hospital.

By 1954 the Oliver Bird Fund promised a further £70,000 to the Manchester Unit and £38,000 had been allocated to Edinburgh for the Rheumatic Unit, to include £27,000 for a new building which was opened in 1955. With increasing money at its disposal an ever widening range of research projects was supported.

The Nuffield Fellowship Programme.

Another important development was the programme of Fellowships in Chronic Rheumatism. In 1948 there were four recipients. They were: Tommy Highton, who later went to New Zealand to work in the rheumatology services in Rotorua and Christchurch; Alan Hill from Edinburgh, later Director of the rheumatology service at Stoke Mandeville Hospital; Robert Moore, later to join Professor Kellgren at Manchester, and Reg Newns, who joined Harry West at Sheffield. In 1949 Bruce Cruikshank and Norrie Swanson, both from Edinburgh, received fellowships. Other Fellowships followed, some from the Foundation and some paid out of the Oliver Bird money.

Increasing wealth.

The £450,000 originally available to the Oliver Bird Fund was supplemented in 1963 when Captain Bird died. He had created a family Trust for his

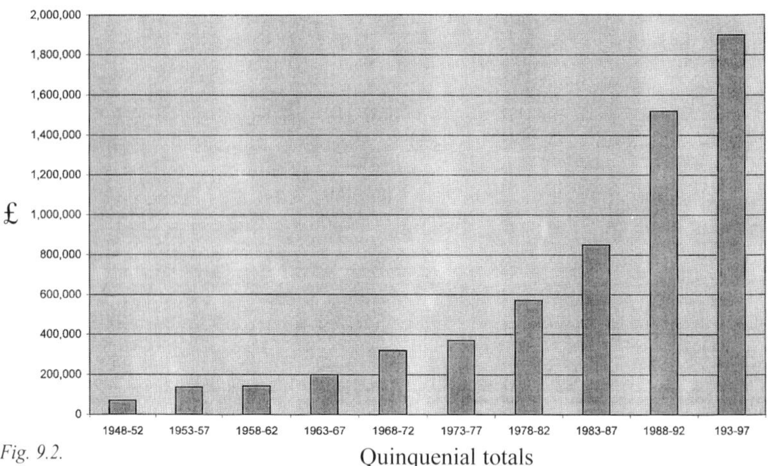

Fig. 9.2.

wife and children but the children did not survive and Mrs Bird renounced her interest in the family trust in favour of the Oliver Bird Fund. He had thus provided the Fund with altogether about £750,000.

With it the Trustees of the Fund performed a modern version of the miracle of the loaves and the fishes. In 1998, as a result of their investment policies, the capital of the fund stood at £12m and in 1997 the Fund was able to spend £468,732 on research, more than the original donation (Fig 9.2). This was celebrated in 1998 by special bursaries and a major scientific conference (Botting and Botting, 1999) to mark the Fund's 50th anniversary.

Welfare Organisations

Arthritis Care

Arthritis Care was founded as the British Rheumatism Association in 1947 by Mr ACN Bowen, an arthritis sufferer. He approached one of the physicians of the Charterhouse Clinics and five Members of Parliament who lent their support, one of them the Minister for Agriculture. In1948 Lord Horder agreed to become Vice-President and negotiated the 'territorial division' so that the Association did not involve itself in research funding and the ARC did not do welfare. In 1949 the two organisations jointly approached the Ministry of Health to propose a regional rheumatism scheme but the co-operation did not last. Sir Stanley Davidson of the ARC felt that the British Rheumatism Association was not sticking to the agreement and in 1950 the liaison committee was dissolved. In 1952 the Association applied to the Board of Trade for incorporation as a public limited liability company but the ARC persuaded the Board to write into the Association's constitution a rule that excluded medical scientific work from its activities. There may have been some bruised egos over this for in 1954 the Association publicly attacked the ARC for not promoting rheumatology rehabilitation services and launched a major appeal for £150,000 headed by Lord Nuffield.

A prominent figure in the early days of the Association was Mrs Neville Rolfe, who was adept at fund-raising events. The finances of the Association went into the red in 1950 but later recovered and at one time rivalled those of ARC. Property acquisition and adaptation supplemented fund raising and lobbying for rheumatism sufferers. In 1950 it formed BRA Homes Ltd and opened a home at Bracken Hill House in Middlesex, but this closed in 1956 for lack of support. Other activities included arranging holidays for otherwise home-bound sufferers and, through its regional network, helping with house maintenance and other activities at home which could not otherwise be provided.

Although not a founder, Dr Francis Bach became involved in the British Rheumatism Association at an early stage and was perceived as its medical champion just as Copeman was the champion of ARC. The initials BRA were considered flippant and the Association changed its name to British Rheumatism and Arthritis Association (BRAA). In the 1970s the name was changed again to Arthritis Care (AC), which upset the ARC because of the similarities of the abbreviations. Arthritis Care now has a 'Young Arthritis' section for members up to the age of 40 and has in the past provided facilities for the support groups for ankylosing spondylitis and for lupus sufferers. For most of the years since 1950 little was done by either Arthritis Care or the ARC to present a common front to the public and politicians. Dr Francis Bach predicted that a merger would never happen as the paid officers of the organisations had vested interests in keeping them apart.

Nevertheless there was a common forum in the British League against Rheumatism (BLAR) and some of the ARC and AC branches co-operated at local level. In 1999 tentative approaches were made by Arthritis Care to explore possible co-operation over the supply of educational material directed at rheumatism sufferers. Other co-operative projects are under discussion.

In order to link with the European League against Rheumatism (EULAR) and thence to the International League against Rheumatism (ILAR) there had to be one single organisation representing each country. The British League against Rheumatism set up in the 1950's became the federal organisation of all societies interested in aspects of the rheumatic diseases. It elected the UK representatives to EULAR and ILAR and for ten years that was its only function. Later it provided a diary of courses and congresses from the ARC's offices. But it was not until the 1980's, under the chairmanship of Professor Maini that it began to represent various groups of the disabled at local level, putting their needs to local health and hospital authorities.

The Horder Homes.

In 1952 Miss Cecilia Bochenek, a small, persuasive and intense woman who had been badly crippled by Juvenile Chronic Arthritis since the age of seven, approached Lord Horder for assistance in setting up a home for arthritics, to teach them how to make the best of their lives. It was to be a sort of convalescent home and re-education facility, a halfway house between hospital and home. There were also to be 'Horder Helpers', people who would volunteer to provide support in the community. Fund raising began, as it did with the ARC, with appeals to the 'great and good' (and rich) but broadened later through a regional organisation. The Marchioness of Dufferyn and Ava, of the Guinness family, was persuaded to give land at Crowborough in Sussex, a decision she is said to have subsequently regretted. A large sum was raised partly as a result of a television appeal and the building was opened in 1961. By 1963 there were 30 regional supporters' groups.

The initiative despite goodwill all round was relatively short lived. Cecilia Bochenek was very much the driving force. Her partner Dr Joyce Peake, nominally the Medical Director, was a weak second in command. The medical aspects of the work were poor. Prof. Bywaters, whose patient Miss Bochenek had been, urged her to get more local medical support. When Dr Peake died Dr Douglas Woolf took over as part time Medical Director and organised a Medical Advisory Committee that included Drs Barbara Ansell and David Doyle and Professors Pat Woo and Rodney Grahame and a representative of the ARC. When Cecilia Bochenek died Dr Douglas Woolf and Ms Dorothy Beaumont worked to upgrade the building and develop it into an orthopaedic centre, which has been successful.

The National Back Pain Association

This partly lay partly medical organisation was founded in 1968 to support research and to educate people in how to alleviate or prevent back problems. It issued manuals for topics such as handling patients and advice on safe lifting. Mr Stanley Grundy, an industrialist, founded it. He was concerned with the extent of back pain ill health in his employees. He favoured chiropractic at first. In the early 1970s the Association sent a representative to the Executive Committee of ARC to try and ensure co-operation, an arrangement which did not last. It helped set up an independent Society for Back Pain Research in 1971, a society of doctors and other health professionals interested in all aspects of the problem and open to heterodox practitioners provided their observations and researches were carried out along scientific lines and the results published at meetings or in the scientific press.

Patient groups in support of rheumatic disease sufferers

Twenty-five societies were listed in the 1997 *Handbook of the British Society for Rheumatology*. They were written to and 18 responded. They were questioned on when their society was set up and by whom, whether they received financial help from the Department of Health, whether they raised money for research and how many members they had. They were asked what other help, apart from more money which every group wanted, they felt they might reasonably expect and what they considered their most important achievements to date. They were also asked to send a copy of their annual accounts from which their current income and surplus (or deficit) could be noted.

Sixteen said which year they were established. Ten started in the decade 1980-89, five earlier than that and one later. Between them [membership numbers in square brackets, where supplied] they covered: arachnoiditis, arthrogryposis [480], Behcet's disease [900], bone dysplasias (two societies), Sjogren's Syndrome [2,200], children's chronic arthritis, dermatomyositis, Ehlers Danlos syndrome [1,500], hypermobility, systemic lupus [3000], Marfan's Syndrome [1,400 families], ankylosing spondylitis [10,000], osteoporosis [23,000], Paget's disease [2,500], Perthe's disease

[1000], psoriatic arthropathy, Raynaud's syndrome plus scleroderma [13,000], restricted growth [700], repetitive strain injury, sarcoidosis [5000 'contacts'], scleroderma (a separate society) [300], scoliosis [2,400], and Wegener's disease.

Doctors set up three of the societies, the rest were established by concerned or affected individuals. There were several instances of apparent duplication of effort. Another hypermobility society existed but was not listed in the *Handbook* and there were two societies for scleroderma.

Eight societies had received a grant from the Department of Health. Almost all wanted greater awareness on the part of the public and the profession of the diagnosis and the problems of their disease. The Psoriatic Arthropathy Alliance and the Scleroderma Societies thought that prescription charges for the ointments they needed should be waived. The help that the Scoliosis Society needed most was to reduce the waiting list for operation, particularly poignant since the longer the wait and the older the child the more difficult the correction of the deformity.

Four societies said they had local groups [numbers]: National Ankylosing Spondylitis Society [100], Lupus UK [29], National Back Pain Association [62], National Osteoporosis Society [50]. Twelve societies gave some money for research but only the larger ones had Scientific Advisory Committees that could ensure best use of the money. Fourteen stated their annual incomes, the total was £4,683,000 but if the four richest were excluded the remaining ten societies shared £1,425,000 between them. Most societies made a surplus during the year. The National Ankylosing Spondylitis Society (NASS) had a net surplus of £50,559 for 1997-8, 80% of which came from legacies.

Societies had been most successful when they had acquired sympathetic guidance from interested specialists. A danger has been a tendency for some of them, dissatisfied with the help they received from their family doctors, to fall under the influence of non-medical practitioners. Some, such as NASS, have formed or joined international affiliations. 'Localism' often led to small breakaway groups.

Their histories followed a pattern exemplified by The National Association for the Relief of Paget's Disease. This was started in 1973 by Mrs Ann Stansfield out of her need to do something to help her husband who had suffered from this bone disease for 27 years and her difficulties in obtaining information and advice. She spent many hours in correspondence with specialists in this country and abroad and at the same time collected together a group of Paget's Disease sufferers. To fund this she and her husband, their friends and the members of the group made cuddly toys and collected gifts and sold them on market stalls. In 1975 she involved the Rehabilitation and Medical Research Trust (now known as 'REMEDI'). The Trust set up a Scientific Advisory Committee of experts in bone diseases for her and for a while took over the management of the money she had collected, including payment of grants for research, until the National Association became independent. The timing was opportune as effective treatments were by then being developed. Medical industry became interested and provided funds for meetings and scientific conferences that sufferers as well as scientists could attend.

By 1998 there were 2,500 members, the disease could be kept under control, there was strong (but disputed) evidence that a canine distemper virus was the cause and a heritability factor had been located on chromosome 18q. The disease had been linked to otosclerosis. Epidemiology had disclosed a concentration of cases in Northwest England. Thanks to successful medical treatment a variety of corrective surgical procedures could be used to overcome the disabilities and deformities caused by the disease.

It is doubtful if advance would have been so rapid without an organised and vocal pressure group.

Reverie

So where has it got us, all this money collected and all this effort by the 'Fourth Estate of Rheumatology'? To parody Browning's 'Grammarian's Funeral':

> *This scientific doctor, aiming for the cure of arthritis, dies ere he knows it.*
>
> *This rehabilitationist, aiming low, achieves a useful gadget.*

Through welfare organisations we can empathise with peoples' problems. With laboratory science we are insulated from them, but might, just might, make medical history. Down which road to go? It is the special perplexity of the physician scientist.

Chapter 10
The search for a science base for rheumatology.

To look for the cause of a disease one first needs an appropriate hypothesis. Unlike cardiology or nephrology, rheumatology had no definable or exclusive organ system on which to base such a hypothesis. The search for a science base for research into the rheumatic diseases has passed through a number of phases.

A hypothesis that was current before the Second World War concerned focal infection. At that time immunisation and vaccination were the only means of countering infectious diseases. In 1902 Almoth Wright had developed vaccines from cultures of chronic infections caused by identified microorganisms. For some forms of inflammatory arthritis such as rheumatoid arthritis there were no identifiable bacterial causes. Frank Billings (1912) evolved an attractive but erroneous hypothesis. He pointed out that we all carry potentially harmful 'passenger' microorganisms in sites from nose to anus. The microorganisms were tolerated because they did not invade the body as a whole even if they were locally responsible for limited areas of sepsis. His suggestion was that when those localised areas of sepsis were associated with other adverse health factors their presence could set off arthritis, nephritis or other pathology.

It must have seemed a logical next step to use autogenous vaccines (i.e. made from the patients 'own' resident bacteria) to treat rheumatoid arthritis. His ideas were taken up uncritically. Autogenous vaccines prepared by Wright at St Mary's Hospital became the mainstays of some private physicians who treated rheumatoid arthritis. The method was particularly associated with Dr Warren Crowe and the Charterhouse Clinics in London. It spread to Belfast in the 1940s and hung on in London until the early 1950s. Following the same reasoning, surgeons removed teeth, tonsils, gall bladders, appendices and piles, even colons in the hope of relieving symptoms.

Billings himself did a comparative trial of autogenous vaccine therapy and found his patients 'did just as well without as with it'. He castigated the proponents of autogenous vaccines in the USA.

"Based on the work of Wright, but disrespectful of the principles developed by him, therapeutic vaccination has progressed in this country into an irrational fad which is intensified and made degrading to the medical profession and harmful to the patients by commercial greed". (Billings, 1916)

The next attempt to create a science base for rheumatology reflected the changing nomenclature. Klemperer (1942) had used the word 'collagen' in the literal sense of 'jelly making'. He conceived the idea that the target tissues in the rheumatic diseases were the collagen fibres with their interstitial ground substance that formed the internal scaffolding of all organs but especially of the locomotor apparatus. Klemperer was an immigrant to the USA and English was not his mother tongue. He called rheumatoid arthritis and related conditions 'collagen diseases', which stimulated research into the chemistry of collagen and interstitial 'ground substance'. Synovial fluid was seen as a specialised form of ground substance since both contained hyaluronic acid. Between the 1969 and 1978 editions of Copeman's 'Textbook of the Rheumatic Diseases' the name was changed from 'collagen diseases' to 'disorders of connective tissue' with equal lack of justification, but that name has stuck. Much early work on collagen that was done in rheumatology research laboratories, such as using an enzyme to remove the polysaccharide elements from skin, is now chiefly of interest to leather chemists. Nevertheless it made an important contribution to the basic biology. Both Bywaters and Kellgen were influenced by Walter Bauer at the Massachusetts General Hospital (MGH) in Boston. Bauer had raised funds to build an arthritis research unit at the Hospital and appointed Drs Jerry Gross and Roger Jeanloz to work on collagen and its associated polysaccharides, respectively. Laboratories at Manchester, Taplow and later the Kennedy Institute followed suit.

Professor David Jackson was the collagen biochemist for ten years in the Manchester Centre for Research into Chronic Rheumatism until 1966. He recalls how he made an accidental discovery. He had prepared a solution of purified collagen but left it on the bench when he was called away. On returning he found that it had turned into a gel. It was on such a gel that Jerry Gross in Boston first demonstrated vertebrate collagenase by culturing a piece of bullfrog tadpole tail on the gel and showing lysis. The Massachusetts General Hospital group later went on to discover human collagenases.

The world wide interest in the chemistry of connective tissues has 'paid off' in embryology and in bone disease, especially osteoporosis, where bone collagen breakdown products are now used to measure the disease and its response to treatment. It came full circle in the study of wound healing and fibrosis.

Wounds on a foetus heal without forming a scar. Starting from this observation Dr Mark Ferguson and others in Manchester have analysed the contribution of the Transforming Growth Factors 1 and 2 to fibrosis in scars, opening the possibility of pharmacological control of fibrosis in contractures of joints and in scleroderma.

Dr Helen Muir was the biochemist and director of the Kennedy Institute who did pioneering work on the proteoglyan aggregates that fill the spaces between collagen fibres and are constituents of cartilage and synovial fluid. She discovered the link protein that held together the proteoglycan sub-units. This opened the way to a better understanding of certain congenital skeletal diseases in which there are abnormalities of proteoglycan metabolism.

After collagen diseases came Selye's 'diseases of stress' and arguments about whether aspirin worked by being adrenocorticotrophic. Then came autoimmunity, then autoimmunity with frills, assuming that some microbial invader by means of a chemical similarity with a body tissue could trigger a response which not only attacked the invader but also the tissue it resembled. There were good grounds for thinking that was what happened in rheumatic fever.

Infection with the *Group A,-haemolytic streptococcus* (GpA,-βHS) had already been discovered to be the trigger that set off rheumatic fever in some but not all children. In 1948 the logical science base for research into rheumatic fever had been the study of the causative microorganism. Work at the Canadian Red Cross Memorial Hospital in Taplow sought to narrow it down to specific sub-types of the streptococcus.

There remained the problem of why some children infected with GpA,-βHS developed rheumatic fever when others did not. An inherited defect in immune responses seemed likely. At that time the study of immunology was in its infancy and the different functions of T- and B-lymphocytes had not been fully unraveled. By 1958 rheumatic fever had almost disappeared so it was no longer a problem. Nevertheless rheumatic fever exemplified the association of an identified environmental factor (infection) together with a host factor (thought to be an inherited predisposition) combining to set off an abnormal host reaction (arthritis) which has served as a model for research into other rheumatic diseases.

Environmental Factor + Host factor = Rheumatic Disease

Figure. 10.1

Those who searched for the causes of rheumatoid arthritis had an even stronger reason to look to immunology. Waaler before 1939 discovered and Rose in 1948 rediscovered that the blood of a rheumatoid arthritis sufferer contained a factor that could agglutinate a suspension of sheep red cells coated with rabbit anti-sheep cell antibody globulin. Globulins were so-called because their molecules were globular in shape. Their involvement in the antibody antigen reaction changed their shape and exposed new reactive sites to which the rheumatoid factors could bind. Rheumatoid factors were thus antibodies to the core of the antibody molecule. A positive Rose-Waaler test had a 90+% correlation with rheumatoid arthritis associated with rheumatoid subcutaneous nodules. This was a higher clinical / laboratory correlation than any other biological tests at the time, such as the Wasserman or Kahn tests for syphilis. Here at last was something that the immunologists could get their teeth into and explore for specificity. In the 1950's, while rheumatology was still struggling to get recognised as a legitimate specialty of medicine, immunology was seized upon as its science base. The British Society for Immunology was set up in 1956 with a number of rheumatologists among its members. Their faith was strengthened when it was shown that thoracic duct drainage, which depletes the body of recycled lymhocytes, could bring about a remission of rheumatoid arthritis. But it was not a practical long-term treatment.

The case for disordered immune functions was even stronger in Systemic Lupus Erythematosis (SLE). The Hargraves (lupus) cell had been discovered (1948) and technological advances clearly showed this was an example of autoimmunity. With the cine-microscope one could see the 'victim ' cell surrounded and destroyed by phagocytes. This was followed by reports of a whole raft of anti-nuclear antibodies in SLE. Series of SLE patients were collected and subjected to repeated investigations. Discovering new antibodies in lupus became like stamp collecting. *How* these antibodies were made has become clearer but *why* they were made still eludes us. None were 100% diagnostically specific although anti-double-stranded DNA was the nearest. The pattern of antinuclear antigens could sometimes predict the clinical manifestations of lupus.

The immunology field was widened by the reports on circulating antigen-antibody-complement complexes in the connective tissue diseases. It was already known that the local injection of an antigen into an animal immunized against that antigen would produce the damaging inflammation of an Arthus reaction. If given intravenously the antibody-antigen combination would cause serum sickness including arthritis. Antibody-antigen complexes were certainly found in blood and tissue sections in rheumatoid arthritis and SLE and related diseases, sometimes in high titres. A whole 'complex industry' grew up. Unfortunately the results of different assay methods did not correlate well with each other nor with clinical manifestations. There were other anomalies. It did not help to measure the complexes circulating in the blood in lupus nephritis since these were not the same as the complexes blocking the capillaries of the glomeruli.

At one time the research interest of most professors of rheumatology in the UK was in lupus immunology or the study of immune complexes and levels of complement. The programmes of the scientific meetings of the Heberden Society in the 1970s reflected this. In 1986 the last edition of Copeman's Textbook of the Rheumatic Diseases devoted 34 pages and 200 references to immune complexes. The 1994 Klippel, Dieppe textbook 'Rheumatology' contained only four lines on immune complexes and the programme of the 1998 meeting of the British Society for Rheumatology (BSR) nothing at all.

The search shifted to immunogenetics, (nine papers at the BSR in 1998). This followed the elucidation of the major histocompatability genes in connection with transplantation research. At the Westminster Hospital the transplantation scientist DCO James had asked his rheumatologist colleagues Hart and Brewerton if they knew of any rheumatic disease that showed strong familial aggregation and might be worth testing with the new leucocyte typing reagents. The answer was 'Yes: ankylosing spondylitis' and the near 100% association of ankylosing spondylitis with the leucocyte antigen HLA B27 was discovered (Brewerton and colleagues 1973). The discovery was made independently by Schlosstein and colleagues (1973) at Los Angeles. An association between another leukocyte antigen, HLA DR4 and rheumatoid arthritis discovered later was not so close (Panayi et al, 1978, Statsny, 1978), although it could rise to near 100% in patients who also had overt vasculitis or Felty's syndrome.

The demonstration of inherited susceptibility to certain rheumatic diseases has broadened to look at many more gene products; in particular those involved in the inflammatory process. The most advanced form of genetic analysis involved genome-wide scanning for linkages to specific rheumatic diseases.

For ankylosing spondylitis and other spondylopathies where the host factor for susceptibility was HLA B27 the environmental precipitating factor could be one of several causes of enterocolitis, including *Yersinia entercolitica, Chlamidia* species, various bacterial causes of dysentery and perhaps other microorganisms. But for rheumatoid arthritis no environmental factor has yet been discovered.

The associations with HLA genotypes have explained some of the geographic differences in the frequency of these diseases There is an increased prevalence of both HLA B27 and ankylosing spondylitis in northern Norway and in countries of the Mediterranean coast of Africa. HLA markers cannot predict what will happen to the individual, since the same genes can occur in unaffected persons. Theorists have speculated that ankylosing spondylitis might be eliminated if all carriers of the HLA B27 gene were sterilised. Quite apart from being unethical such a proposal would not work. The disease is usually not detected until after the sufferer has become sexually active. Moreover clinical experience and acquaintance with the membership of the National Ankylosing Spondylitis Society shows that this disease is not infrequently associated with high achievement. Included amongst those affected are artists, musicians, leading members of the professions and captains of industry. It is possible that the HLA B27 gene confers benefits as well as risks.

Osteoarthritis, in contrast to rheumatoid arthritis, has attracted relatively little scientific exploration. It was originally known as 'degenerative joint disease' and considered to be the result of wear and tear. It was also known as 'hypertrophic arthritis', recognising that central joint wear was associated with marginal joint overgrowth. Bennett and Bauer (1937) published experimental studies on rabbits. They dislocated the patella to the side of the femoral condyle without opening the joint and allowed the animal to run freely. The central articular cartilage of the femur became atrophic although no longer in apposition. At the same time there was rapid wear where the patella moved over the medial aspect of the condyle. This was associated paradoxically with marginal cartilage overgrowth and osteophyte formation on the side of the joint opposite the dislocation of the patella. Today we would interpret this as the release into the joint of a specific, locally active, cartilage growth factor that has yet to be identified.

There is a female preponderance of the nodal form of osteoarthritis that was distinguished by Kellgren and Moore (1952) and certain other patterns of osteoarthritis tend to run in families, suggesting genetic predispositions. In pursuit of this, Arthritis Research Campaign-supported work at Oxford (Prof. Brian Smith and colleagues) has screened the entire genome of 481 families in order to find the genes or combinations of genes that might be responsible.

Because osteoarthritis had been considered to be a purely degenerative joint disease attempts were made to call it osteo*arthrosis*, i.e. non-inflammatory. But Hutton and others (1986) showed by thermography and scintigraphy that inflammation and increased bone turnover preceded the appearance of osteoarthritis in the terminal interphalangeal joints and the name osteo*arthritis* has been accepted.

Radin and his co-workers (1991) have explored impact absorption in the larger weight bearing joints. They found that the denser and less elastic the bone the more likely it was to transmit excess impact forces to articular cartilage, leading to cartilage breakdown. While this could hardly explain all osteoarthritis, particularly that of the small joints of the fingers, it fitted in well with other observations. Femoral heads removed at operation for osteoporotic fractures of the neck of femur seldom showed osteoarthritis, while osteoarthritic hips seldom suffered a fracture of the neck of the femur.

Studies on the aetiology of osteoarthritis have been overshadowed by the success of orthopaedic surgeons in devising mechanical solutions for the pain and disability that it has causes. For thirty years, until about 1965, the McMurray osteotomy of the hip had been the standard treatment for hip disease. It relieved pain in osteoarthritis 'Although how it worked was a mystery' (Waugh, 1993). Wedge osteotomies of the knee were used for varus (bow-legged) and valgus (knock-knee) deformities. They relieved pain and improved gait. A more radical approach to osteoarthritis was to replace the whole joint by a permanent biocompatible metal prosthesis. The problem was more straightforward for the hip, a ball and socket joint, although a suitable prosthesis took years to perfect. Getting there involved metallurgy, materials science and adhesives technology. Its success is particularly linked to the name of John Charnley. For the knee, a constrained hinge joint, the difficulties were greater and many different designs were developed.

Drilling of exposed eburnated articular bone in osteoarthritic knees in the 1960s showed that fibrocartilage could regenerate from the drill holes although not of sufficient quality to be clinically useful. Nevertheless it pointed to the possibility of healing in this disease. By 1997 knowledge of cartilage morphogenetic and growth factors had improved to the extent that articular cartilage cells could be taken from a biopsy and multiplied in culture in a form that appeared to be suitable for resurfacing cartilage defects ('*Times*', 1998).

Early work on the physiology of joints that had been done at the Massachusetts General Hospital compared the exchange of various crystalloids and colloids between the joint fluid and the blood in the resting joint. But joints are structures moving under power and their normal and morbid physiology needs to be assessed in that context. The pressure in a resting knee is sub-atmospheric and falls further during walking. The pressure gradient in the normal knee reduces from bone to cartilage and from capsule to synovium, favouring the flow of nutrients into the joint. Enormous pressures, over a metre of mercury, could be generated in the synovial fluid of a knee that was used when distended by fluid (Dixon and Grant, 1965), and the pressure gradients were reversed. Irrespective of the diagnostic label of the arthritis, this could lead to acute and chronic synovial rupture, juxta-articular synovial cysts and the extrusion of synovial fluid and hypertrophied synovium through erosions into bone ends, recognised on X-ray as 'geodes'. In the knee those pressures caused reflex inhibition of the quadriceps muscles (Dixon and Hawkins, 1989). It made no more sense to study the resting joint than it would to study cardiac physiology by stopping the heart.

The equivalent in the joints of stopping the heart is paralysis of a limb. The clinical manifestations of rheumatoid arthritis do not occur, or are much diminished, in limbs paralysed before the onset of the arthritis. This led to speculation about a neurogenic cause for rheumatoid arthritis. However the phenomenon is also seen in osteoarthritis and in both lower and upper motor neurone causes of paralysis, (reviewed in Dixon and Hawkins,1989). Prof. David Blake when at the Royal London Hospital, from 1987-97, has extended this work to study the effects of high intra-articular pressures in compressing synovial capillaries and causing intermittent synovial ischaemia. In doing so he has opened up a new basis for research in arthritis.

Blake (1998) questioned *in vitro* immunology research that had not taken into account the oxygen stress that could obtain in the inflamed joint. The rheumatoid synovium was stuffed with T-lymphocytes, often seen as the villains of the piece and the cause of joint destruction, but he did not consider it likely that they would function in vivo as they did when oxygen replete in vitro. Blake believed it to be more likely that the macrophage/fibroblast system was upregulated and might be a better target for research into ways of healing inflammatory arthritis. His theories were disputed by some of his colleagues, who considered that T-lymphocytes were important in the pathogenesis of rheumatoid arthritis and that they acted in concert with the macrophage/ fibroblast system in producing the final picture of the disease.

The study of arthritis in animals has made contributions although differences in size and body weight made it insecure to extrapolate from experimental animals to the human animal. LE Glynn pointed out that the laboratory rabbit was amongst the most idle of creatures. If active use of a joint modified the expression of disease in that joint the study of that animal had limitations.

However, Glynn's collagen arthritis in rabbits and Freund's adjuvant arthritis in rats did play a part in the ARC-funded development of Anti-tumour Necrosis Factor- therapy in rheumatoid arthritis and this has opened a new door to possibilities of treatments. Experimental animal models have not told us much about the way that anti-rheumatoid arthritis drugs such as gold or penicillamine work. The standard animal model of osteoarthritis, made by cutting the cruciate ligaments of the dog, has alerted us to the inevitable damage in man if ruptured cruciates are not promptly mended.

A search for naturally-occurring animal analogues of human inflammatory rheumatic diseases has so far been relatively fruitless. A dog with a naturally occurring analogue of human rheumatoid arthritis complete with nodules and positive tests for rheumatoid factor has been described but 'research is hampered by animal rights issues' (Panayi). A form of chronic arthritis in monkeys was discovered in 1981. Despite the millions of animals bred or killed for their hides and pelts, none have been seen with generalised scleroderma although localised scleroderma (morphea) has been recorded in a dog and in a cat. Laboratory models of scleroderma include the 'tight-skin mouse' (Black, 1999). Animal analogues of systemic lupus, either naturally occurring or experimentally induced, do exist in mice, mink and dogs and have extended the science base of lupus. Haemophilia and osteogenesis imperfecta occur in dogs and hypertrophic pulmonary osteoarthropathy has been recorded in a wide variety of mammalian species. Gout occurs in some birds when fed on high protein diets but the mechanism is different.

Much research funded by the ARC or the Oliver Bird Fund is not targeted directly at named human rheumatic diseases. It investigates the basic processes of inflammation, immunity, immune tolerance and genetics. It has to be seen against an enormous world wide thrust by both academic and commercial laboratories into areas being revealed by the new genetics and made possible by inventions affecting analysis, synthesis and manufacture such as the polymerase chain reaction.

The commonest complaint dealt with by rheumatologists is back pain and here the search for a unifying explanation has been the least rewarding. A valid science base would indicate ways of preventing back pain. But there are many causes of back pain, not all of them arising in the back. Some degree of intervertebral disc degeneration seems inevitable with age. Hutton suggested, unhelpfully, that mankind was badly engineered for its evolution to bipedal upright locomotion. Biochemists have done extensive studies on the hydration and chemistry of the intervertebral discs. Anatomists have pointed out that impingement on nerve roots depends not only on the size of disc protrusions but critically on the size and shape of the spinal canal into which they protrude. It took the advent of magnetic resonance imaging to prove that compression of veins in the intervertebral foramina could cause congestion and oedema of the nerve roots leading to pain in the back and referred pain in the nerve root territory. Could this have been more widely known earlier? Bradford and Spurlings' monograph on the intervertebral disc (See Chapter 8. Page 113) illustrated nerve root oedema in 1927, although they did not relate it to venous congestion.

Progress in back pain research will depend on better means of diagnosis. Advanced forms of ultrasonic imaging look promising. And doubtless there will be surgical approaches to the minority of attacks of back pain that do not spontaneously improve with the passage of time. Meanwhile the waters are muddied by the host of practitioners that Brian Inglis (1964) has classed as 'Fringe medicine' [19], most of whom claim to improve or cure back troubles by their particular approach.

Chapter 11
Professional communication

Professional communication in rheumatology in the United Kingdom could be said to have started in 1935 with the *Reports on Chronic Rheumatic Diseases* that in 1939 became the *Annals of Rheumatic Diseases.* It was planned at the British Red Cross Clinic for Rheumatism in Peto Place, Marylebone, in London.

The Red Cross Clinic had been opened in 1930 and was the first outside the spa hospitals to offer deep pool exercises for arthritics. There were also a number of methods of delivering passive heat. Its treatments were cheap and for the moneyless were subsidised. It was popular with patients and with doctors who wanted to come and study the methods and the diseases treated. Fig. 11.1 shows the staffing structure and management in 1946 when it was decided to employ a medical registrar (one of these was Dr Douglas Woolf) in order to lighten the load on the voluntary consultants and facilitate more teaching. Dr Woolf describes how, while he got on with the work, the consultants would visit, smoke, drink tea and discuss. It was in 1936 that six physicians of the Clinic formed the 'Committee for the Study and Investigation of Rheumatism' that in 1937 became the Heberden Society.

Selected members of the Society formed the Howitt Club, a dining club where plans were made for the future of rheumatology and physical medicine.

On the left of Figure 11.1 are listed the visiting physicians, most of them well known names whose contributions to rheumatology are recounted in Moll's *The Heberden Society*. Kersley from Bath and Patterson from Droitwich took the more disabled patients to the spas. Miss Doris Baker may be remembered by some for her description of the 'Panniculitis of Doris Baker,' the tender fatty swellings that could affect the medial side of the knee in overweight women. Horace Turney and Kenneth Stone were older style physical medicine doctors who also did rheumatic disease clinics.

Early meetings of the Society were held in the Red Cross Clinic. As the Society grew it needed ever larger premises for its scientific meetings that were held twice a year, one in London and one in the hospital of doctor nominated as the Heberden Roundsman. Giving the Heberden Round was an honour but also an opportunity to inform a wider audience about the Roundsman's approach to treatment and research. (Table 11.1 lists the names of the Roundsmen from last to first).

The library of the British Medical Association lists fifteen peer-reviewed journal titles in rheumatology. The *Annals of Rheumatic Diseases* was the official journal of both the British and North American rheumatology societies until 1958 when the American *Arthritis and Rheumatism* was started. The *Annals of Physical Medicine* followed in 1952. It published an increasing numbers of papers on chronic rheumatic diseases until its content was similar to that of the *Annals*. In 1972 it was renamed *Rheumatology and Rehabilitation.*

When the Heberden Society was absorbed into the British Society for Rheumatology in 1984 the tradition of the Heberden Round was continued but there was a problem as to which should be the official journal. The British Medical Association owned the *Annals of Rheumatic Diseases* but offered terms less good than those of the

CLINIC FOR RHEUMATISM

Committee of Management:

C. G. Izard, Esq., O.B.E. (*Chairman*)

W. S. C. Copeman, Esq., O.B.E., M.D., F.R.C.P.
R. H. W. Hope, Esq., O.B.E., M.C.
F. D. Howitt, Esq., C.V.O., M.D., F.R.C.P.
Henry Lesser, Esq., O.B.E., LL.B.
Sir Frederick Menzies, K.B.E., M.D., F.R.C.P.
A. M. A. Moore, Esq., F.R.C.S.
F. H. D. Pritchard, Esq.
M. B. Ray, Esq., O.B.E., D.S.O., M.D., M.R.C.P.
W. S. Tegner, Esq., M.B., M.R.C.P.
Air-Marshal Sir Harold Whittingham, K.C.B., K.B.E.,
Mrs. Williams-Ellis, J.P.
The Lady Woolton.

Administrator: H. Gordon Thompson, Esq., M.D., F.R.C.S.

Honorary Consulting Physicians:

Sir William Hale-White, K.B.E., M.D., F.R.C.P.
The Rt. Hon. Lord Horder, G.C.V.O., M.D., F.R.C.P.
Professor Sir Leonard Hill, M.B., F.R.S.
Sir Frederick Menzies, K.B.E., M.D., F.R.C.P.
Sir Edward Stewart, K.B.E., M.D., M.R.C.P.

Visiting Medical Staff and Medical Board:

M. B. Ray, Esq., O.B.E., D.S.O., M.D., M.R.C.P.
F. D. Howitt, Esq., C.V.O., M.D., F.R.C.P.
C. B. Heald, Esq., C.B.E., M.D., F.R.C.P.
W. S. C. Copeman, Esq., O.B.E., M.D., F.R.C.P.
Miss Doris Baker, M.D., M.R.C.P.
H. F. Turney, Esq., M.D., M.R.C.P.
Kenneth Stone, Esq., M.D., M.R.C.P.
E. Fletcher, Esq., M.D., M.R.C.P.
W. S. Tegner, Esq., M.B., M.R.C.P.
J. W. T. Patterson, Esq., M.D., F.R.C.P.
G. D. Kersley, Esq., M.D., F.R.C.P.
Assistant Physician: Oswald Savage, Esq., O.B.E., M.R.C.P
Surgeon: A. M. A. Moore, Esq., F.R.C.S.
Orthopædic Surgeons:
S. L. Higgs, Esq., M.B., F.R.C.S.
W. Coltart, Esq., M.B., F.R.C.S.
Laryngologist: C. Hamblen-Thomas, Esq., F.R.C.S.
Gynæcologist: Miss Lilian Raftery, M.R.C.O.G., M.M.S.A.
Neurologist: J. Purdon Martin, Esq., M.D., F.R.C.P.
Radiologist: F. C. Golding, Esq., M.R.C.P., D.M.R.E.
Assistant Radiologist: Mrs. Helen M. Harper, M.B., B.Ch., D.M.R.E.
Dental Surgeon: Eric E. Wookey, Esq., L.D.S., R.C.S.
Pathologist: J. W. Shackle, Esq., M.A., M.B., B.Ch.

Dermatologist: G. B. Mitchell Heggs, Esq., O.B.E., M.D., F.R.C.P.

Matron:
Miss W. M. McAllister, M.B.E., D.N. (LOND.), C.S.P., S.R.N.

Lady Almoner:
Miss M. W. Edminson, A.I.H.A.

Fig 11.1. The Staff of the Red Cross Clinic for Rheumatism. From the Clinic's Annual Report, 1946

Oxford University press which owned *Rheumatology and Rehabilitation.* The latter was chosen and renamed *The British Journal of Rheumatology (BJR).* This decision offended some past loyalties but the *BJR* grew to have an international face. [Figure 11.2] and in 1999 was renamed *Rheumatology.*

Undergraduate and postgraduate education, textbooks, meetings, conferences and congresses have all changed from a trickle to a tide in 50 years. In the

1960s undergraduate education in rheumatology was interpreted by some medical schools as a visit to a physical medicine department or a Spa hospital, thus Bristol students were taken to Bath. But elsewhere patients with chronic rheumatic diseases with all their medical and social complications were seen as valuable teaching material for students and part of their education in general medicine.

Medical Postgraduate Centres were set up in the 1960s and spread to all District General Hospitals. They were staffed by postgraduate tutors and trained librarians with both traditional and modern information technologies available although these did not displace specialist textbooks. The first (1948) edition of Copeman's *Textbook of the Rheumatic Diseases* weighed $1^1/_2$ Kg. By 1969 the fourth edition weighed 2 $^1/_2$ Kg, the fifth 3kg and in 1984 the sixth and last weighed 5Kg in two

Heberden Roundsman 1948-99

1999 Prof. M DOHERTY
Nottingham

1998 Prof. M I V JAYSON
Manchester

1997 Dr S ROBERTS.
Belfast

1996 Dr M H SEIFERT
London

1995 Dr T E HOTHERSALL
Stoke-on-Trent

1994 Prof. P J MADDISON
Bath

1993 Dr B L HAZLEMAN
Cambridge

1992 Dr M CAWLEY
Southampton

1991 Dr A G MOWAT
Oxford

1990 Dr I GRIFFITHS
Newcastle-upon-Tyne

1989 Dr M SNAITH
London

1988 Prof. P BACON
Birmingham

1987 Dr E C HUSKISSON
London

1986 Dr B BRESNIHAN
Dublin

1985 Dr LENNOX HOLT
Manchester

1984 Prof. P D DIEPPE
Bristol

1983 Prof. G NUKI
Edinburgh

1982 Dr G R V HUGHES
Hammersmith

1981 Dr A M DENMAN
Northwick Park

1980 Dr H W BALME
London

1979 Dr J A COSH
Bath

1978 Dr LOGIE BAIN
Aberdeen

1977 Dr K N LLOYD
Cardiff

1976 Prof. WW BUCHANAN
Glasgow

1975 Dr N CARDOE
Norwich

1974 Dr E B D HAMILTON
London

1973 Prof. V WRIGHT
Leeds

1972 Dr H L F CURREY
London

1971 Dr J T SCOTT
London

1970 Dr W R M
ALEXANDER
Edinburgh

1969 Dr A St J DIXON
Bath

1968 Dr C F HAWKINS
Birmingham

1967 Dr B M ANSELL
Taplow

1966 Dr R M MASON
London

1965 Dr J. SHARP
Buxton

1964 Prof. G A SMART and
Dr M THOMPSON
Newcastle-upon-Tyne

1963 Dr H F WEST
Sheffield

1962 Dr A G S HILL
Stoke Mandeville

1961 Dr 0 SAVAGE
London

1960 Dr W S TEGN ER
London

1959 Prof. E G L
BYWATERS
Hammersmith

1958 Prof. J H GOSLINGS
Leiden

1957 Dr J J R DUTHIE
Edinburgh

1956 Dr G D KERSLEY
Bath.

1955 Dr F DUDLEY HART
London

1954 Prof. S J HARTFALL
Leeds

1953 Prof. J H KELLGREN
Manchester

1952 Prof. Sir H COHEN
Liverpool

1951 Prof. Sir S DAVIDSON
Edinburgh

1950 Prof. F COSTE
Paris

1949 Prof. I.J WITTS
Oxford

1948 Sir L WHITBY
Cambridge

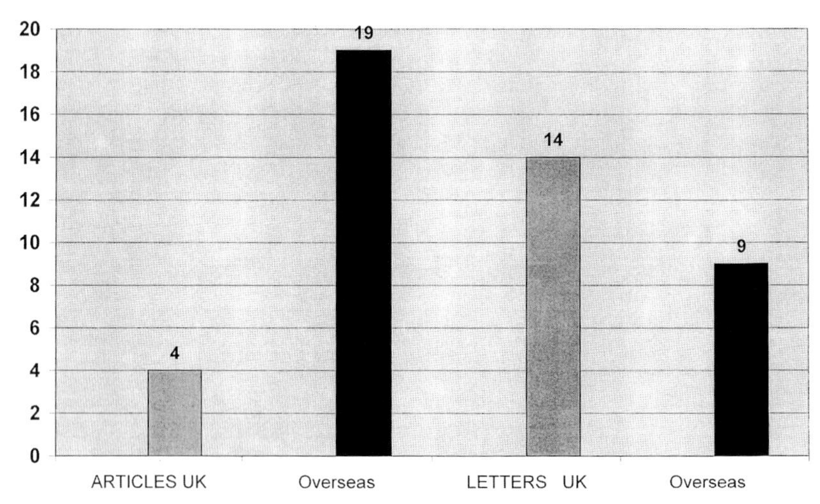

Fig 11.2. British Journal of Rheumatology in 1998, overseas and domestic sources of published articles and letters

volumes. This was topped in 1994 by the massive Klippel- Dieppe *Rheumatology* at 5 1/2 Kg. in a single volume.

In 1948 the membership of the Heberden Society was limited to one hundred. By 1998 there were three thousand in the British Society for Rheumatology. Originally all papers submitted were presented orally, a 'beauty parade ' for young aspiring rheumatologists to show their style.

As the numbers of papers increased committees were set up to select those worthy of oral presentation. To guard against academic nepotism abstracts had to be submitted without the authors' names. In time even this method of reducing the numbers became inadequate, particularly as obtaining expenses to go to a conference might depend on having a letter to say that a paper had been accepted. In some conferences papers were accepted but grouped by topic and the conclusions read out by a raconteur. Today all but small meetings use posters as a way of accommodating the flood of information. Medical illustration became a vital part of professional communication, oral presentations being reserved for well-known figures at plenary sessions to review interesting topics.

Much communication between different departments in a hospital was in the form of 'coffee housing' when doctors met casually for a meal or a tea break or a drink at the end of the day and generally talked shop. It could be contended that the growth of private practice diminished the amount of informal contacts that occurred within the Health Service in this way. Consultants increasingly used the lunch hour for their private work or lunched at their private hospital.

Other contacts occurred at committees. Until about 1950 the Health Service seemed to have unlimited funds. Budget controls were few. Expenditure regularly exceeded estimates. In 1950 a ceiling on NHS expenditure was imposed and

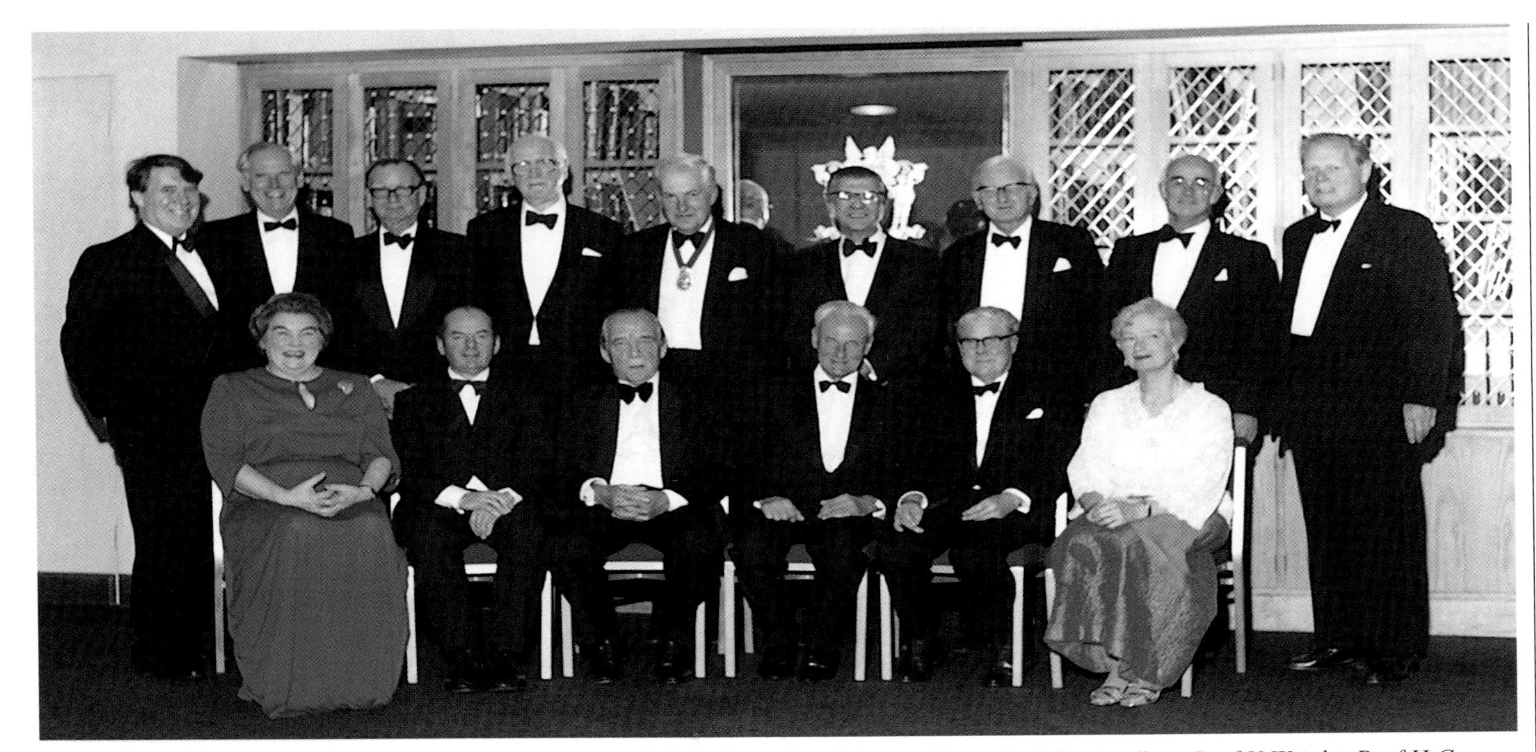

Fig 11.3. Presidents of the Heberden Society who attended the last official dinner. From the left, standing, *Prof V Wright, Prof H Currey, Prof EGL Bywaters, Prof Sir Ronald Tonbridge, Prof D Brewerton, Prof K Walton, Dr C Hawkins, Dr JT Scott, Dr FD Hart.* Sitting, *Dr BM Ansell, Dr AS Dixon, Prof JJR Duthie, Prof JH Kellgren, Dr A Hill, Dr AH Muir.*

plans for new developments met resistance for lack of funds. Choices, often divisive, had to be made in committees.

Hospital committees multiplied both in number and the hours they occupied. They were an unpaid burden on their time for consultants with private practices to see to, for dedicated academics wanting to get on with writing their research papers or simply for those doctors who valued their private time with their families or hobbies.

Yet as Dr Alan Hill when at Stoke Mandeville Hospital said, 'You can never afford to miss a committee- if you do, something you do not want may be decided'. In chapter 4 it was noted how in Glasgow Watson Buchanan's committee-phobia could lead to a disaster which ended with his emigration to Canada.

Of it, he has written-

'In 1977, I happened to notice late one afternoon that the last item of the Glasgow Royal Infirmary Staff Meeting was a proposal to close the Centre for Rheumatic Diseases. I had not intended to go to the meeting, but did so that afternoon. I should say that I have always hated such meetings, wasting hours taking minutes is not my cup of tea. When I got there I was horrified that the issue had already been decided.'

In all regions of the UK from the 1960's on, local rheumatology societies were set up where staff and trainees could meet to exchange ideas, present cases and to review each others' research papers. These meetings acted as rehearsals for national or international conferences. Local clinical societies made it possible to hear what was going on in other disciplines. Teaching hospitals and most District General hospitals had weekly 'Grand Rounds' to which attendance was expected.

The profession paid for some aspects of this professional communication. Other funding came from postgraduate education budgets and drug companies. The latter benefited from an opportunity for their representatives to display and discuss their products.

So where did the ' Drug Reps' get their knowledge? Fifty years ago it was an all male job, and the 'Reps' were little more than salesmen, calling at hospitals and surgeries hoping to get an interview with the doctor, offering samples and executive toys to make this more likely. Today most are women, perhaps recruited from medically related jobs such as nursing or pharmacy. Others may have studied biochemistry, but all will have been put through a brief but intensive educational programme by their employers, aimed at improving knowledge of the products they are to promote and grilling them on how to answer the questions doctors will most likely ask.

The changes in the National Health Service since 1948 were accompanied by increasing liberalisation of attitudes among its workers. Rigid demarcations between family doctors and hospital consultants softened. Whereas before the war consorting with an unregistered practitioner was a professional offence that could bring down the wrath of the General Medical Council and the penalty of being struck off the medical register, today cooperation between doctors and complementary medicine in one of its many forms is common. Better knowledge of the treatments for the rheumatic diseases and the waiting list barriers to hospital specialists have inspired the setting up of the Primary Care Rheumatology Society under the leadership of Dr John Dixon and others. By 1999 it had 350 members. It arranged training in rheumatology for primary care physicians by primary care physicians who perhaps understood the practicalities of general practice better than the hospital based consultants. It established protocols for the treatment of named rheumatic diseases and osteoporosis in primary care. It organised a course of training in the University of Bath leading to a diploma in musculoskeletal medicine

Rheumatology nursing has undergone an analogous change. Before the war, patients in hospitals were expected to be in beds with sheets tightly tucked in. Bed cages had to be introduced because this led to pressure sores on heels and elsewhere. By the end of the century patients, especially rheumatic disease patients, were expected to be up and dressed wherever possible. Older nurses had been taught to do everything for their patients but this discouraged self-help and independence. For rheumatology patients, nurses had to learn to do as little as possible yet to stand by and offer help only if needed- a lesson very hard for some to learn if they were in a hurry, but essential if patients were not to be institutionalised by default. In the 1980s courses for rheumatology nursing were organised.

Some nurses provided outreach services of hospital rheumatology departments. They supervised courses of treatment in the home, such as gold injections or immunosuppressives that required regular monitoring of blood and urine tests and liaised with the practice nurses of the primary care health centres. Some nurses, physiotherapists and other health professionals took on the job of monitoring clinical trials of treatments, assuring quality control of the data. Radiographers learnt to measure bone density in osteoporosis patients and progressed from there to running a telephone counseling service. To ensure interprofessional communication, the 'British Health Professionals in Rheumatology' was set up, sharing office accommodation with the British Society for Rheumatology (BSR) and having its own independent conference alongside that of the BSR.

Government and press, conscious of increasing National Health Service costs, have exhorted their citizens and readers to take more personal responsibility for their health. Traditionally people obtained their health information from the local chemist if they did not want to go to the doctor. Others went to 'Health food shops'. The responses of those shops to a standard test list of symptoms which might indicate a brain tumour and the remedies they offered were inconsistent and some were potentially dangerous (Vickers, Rees and Robin, 1998). There was also a flood of health information from television, popular magazines and newspapers of widely varying accuracy. At one end of the spectrum was Dr Thomas Stuttaford of the 'Times' writing articles on topical themes such as an illness in a public figure. At the other end were articles that were little more than a commercially inspired 'plug' for a patent medicine.

Most women's magazines did have an informed author to write articles on women's health issues such as arthritis or osteoporosis. Books on rheumatism were available at libraries and bookshops but for every book based on evidence and current knowledge there might be ten others that claimed to have *the* answer to all rheumatic problems. The medical profession had a constant battle to set the record straight. In this it has been helped by the explanatory leaflets issued by the medical charities and patient support groups that exist for almost every rheumatic disease.

The fax machine, E-mail, telephone link-ups and the Internet are increasingly used for professional communication and will doubtless play an ever larger part in the future.

The phenomenal growth of electronic communication in the 20th century is put in perspective when it is recalled that the British Broadcasting Corporation did not start its services until 1922.

Chapter 12
Drugs, Procedures and Clinical Trials

"The treatment of rheumatoid arthritis does not just come out of a bottle of tablets"
–Walter Bauer, 1954.

Appliances and adaptations and activities of daily living.

It may make more sense for a patient with painful deformed feet to be fitted with comfortable bespoke shoes than to be given the latest pain-killer tablets. Similarly it may be preferable to supply easily graspable cutlery with soft large-diameter neoprine handles rather than resort to hand surgery for a patient with a weak grip who would be unable otherwise to feed herself. The Arthritis Research Campaign, recognising this, in 1999 produced an excellent illustrated booklet listing appliances for the disabled that were both commercially available and 'user tested'.

Patients with chronic rheumatic diseases suffer pain on movement but they also complain of fatigue and the frustration of not being able to get things done. Sometimes even the effort of standing at the sink and washing up is too much.

Dr Frank Cooksey at King's College Hospital transformed much of modern occupational therapy. Hand looms and trays of jigsaw puzzles to while away the time for patients nursed in bed gave place to adaptations of the home and workplace for the needs of the disabled. Aids to daily living were developed. If one could describe a disability there was almost certainly a way of helping overcome the handicap it would cause. Stair lifts, walking aids, powered wheel chairs and adaptations to cars restored mobility. There were libraries of household aids that helped with cooking, toileting, bed making, dressing and communication. Many had been developed at the Mary Marlborough Lodge in Oxford, supported by the Disabled Living Foundation. But arthritis sufferers also required medicines to kill pain and hold the disease in check

The Salicylates

Before 1948 the only practical anti-inflammatory drug for the inflammatory rheumatic diseases was aspirin (acetylsalicylic acid). It was easy for industrial chemists to make in a highly purified state. It was effective and prescribed for all forms of arthritis. Early textbooks suggested it should be given almost to the point of toxicity in children with rheumatic fever. In the USA aspirin treatment was always described as 'mandatory' for rheumatoid arthritis and given in doses of up to 18 x 300mg tablets a day, controlled by salicylate blood levels. Adverse effects included gastro-intestinal bleeding, deafness, tinnitus and fluid retention.

Aspirin had been preceded by sodium salicylate with similar properties. In this country the parent glycoside salicin from which salicylate was derived was extracted from *Filipendula ulmaria* or Meadowsweet. (A modern flora [Philips R, 1977] gives this recipe: 'Filipendula has the same properties as aspirin: steep 45g of the dried flowers in 2 litres of near boiling water for ten minutes. The dose is three cupfuls between meals a day). Salicin was later discovered in *Salix, Populus and Gaulthonia* species. Salicylic acid was made by hydrolysis of salicin in 1835 and synthesised in

1860. The Bayer Company introduced aspirin, acetylsalicylic acid, in 1899 and the name is still their trademark. By 1948 there was already a large body of knowledge about the many properties of aspirin and that year saw the publication of the 'Bible of the Salicylates', (Gross and Greenberg, 1948). By 1962 at the time of the ERC-sponsored International Symposium on Salicylates aspirin was a popular home remedy, swallowed by the public in tonnage quantities for everything from colds to hangovers. Many glorified proprietary brands of aspirin were produced backed by persuasive and often fraudulent claims and sold at prices twenty times that of Aspirin BP.

Studies that used radio-chromium labeling of red cells at Hammersmith Hospital from 1958-61 did not find any marked advantage to any of them as regards gastrointestinal bleeding although the enteric coated and soluble preparations were possibly less liable to cause dyspepsia. In an acid milieu both aspirin and salicylate were subject to non-ionic diffusion which meant that absorption and excretion were strongly influenced by the pH of the gastric juice and of the urine. Aspirin's only rivals were amidopyrine and phenacetin but these lost favour because they could cause renal damage and sometimes bone marrow suppression.

Newer non-steroidal anti-inflammatory agents.

The first new non-steroidal anti-inflammatory drug, or NSAID (pronounced En-Sade) was phenylbutazone. It was marketed in 1951 and supplanted by oxyphenbutazone in 1959. It was remarkably effective in ankylosing spondylitis sufferers for whom it is still prescribable. It was withdrawn from other indications because of a bad record of causing stomach ulcers. There were also rare but worrying instances of fatal agranulocytosis and aplastic anaemia.

The next to be introduced was indomethacin in 1962. It was first available in the UK as tablets that caused adverse gastrointestinal effects. These were less of a problem when the drug was presented in gelatine capsules. Indomethacin could cause drug-induced headache and occasionally psychedelic hallucinations but was less likely than phenylbutazone to cause fluid retention.

There followed a spate of new and supposedly safer or more effective NSAIDs. Table 12.1 lists 63 proprietary preparations in 22 chemical classes. There was no single drug that was outstanding in efficacy or safety but it was useful to have a choice to offer because of patients' preferences and idiosyncrasies. All were launched with media hype as though they were Wonder Drugs. *(One wondered if they were really different and one wondered why they were so expensive!).*

The prize for a company that produced a popular and effective NSAID was so high that some were tempted, perhaps through rogue marketing departments rather than their medical and research departments, to suppress adverse findings when the drug was put out for clinical use. Ely Lilly was accused in a well researched television programme of launching the drug Opren (benoxyprofen) in the UK in the winter of 1980 (a time of low UV light intensity) when it already knew from its experience in the USA that the drug could cause serious and persistent sun-sensitisation. In the elderly, it could cause death from renal failure. This scandal lead to the insistence by the Medicines Commission on all new drugs being specifically tested in the elderly.

Substituted carboxylic acids

Salicylic acids

Aspirin
Solprin
Paynocil
Nu-seals
Onadox
Levius
Laboprin
Hypon
Codis

Antoin
Breoprin
Caprin
Claradin
Aloxiprin
Palaprin
Benorylate
Benoral
Diflunisal
Dolobid
Salsalate
Disalcid
Choline Magnesium Trisalicylate
Trilisate

Propionic acids
Fenbufen
Lederfen

Fenoprofen
Progesic
Fenopron

Flurbiprofen
Froben

Propionic acids (cont.)

Ibuprofen
Brufen
Ebufac
Ibu-slo
Apsifen
Fenbid
Lidifen
Motrin
Paxofen

Ketoprofen
Orudis
Alrheumat
Naproxen
Naprosyn
Napsalgesic
Synflex
Laraflex
Tiaprofenic acid
Surgam
Suprofen
Suprol
Fenamic acids
Mefenamic acid
Ponstan

Benzotriazene
Azapropazone
Rheumox

Enolic acids

Pyrazolones
Feprazone
Methrazone
Phenylbutazone
Butazolidin
Parazoliadin
Butacote

Oxicams
Piroxicam
Feldene
Larapam

Tenoxicam
Imadyl
Phenylacetic acids
Diclofenac
Voltarol
Rhumalgen
Meloxicam
Mobic

Carbo and hetero cyclic acetic acids

Indomethacin
Imbrilon
Indocid
Mobilan
Artracin
Indolar
Nadoflex
Indoflex
Rheumacin
Flexin Continus
Sulindac

Alkamone
Nabumetone
Reliflex
Pyranocarboxylic acids
Etodolac
Lodine
Ramodar

Table 12.1
Non-steroidal anti inflammatory drugs (COX-1 and COX-2 inhibitors)
Chemical groups in italics.
Generic names in bold
Proprietory names in normal style.

Alclofenac, which had been shown in Bath to cause serious skin rashes with systemic upset, had been put to the Medicines Commission as causing no more skin problems than placebos, as a result of a trial run by a clinical testing laboratory in South Wales. Permission had already been given for the drug to be marketed. Rashes were seen in the first study on which the permission was based but in filling in the trial report forms these rashes had been equated with the harmless 'bosom blushes' and mild erythemas that were always recorded with any placebo. Despite warnings from Bath, the company persisted with promoting and marketing until forced by the tide of complaints to withdraw. The moral that should be drawn is that clinical researchers should not undertake trials when the decision to market had already been made, because the findings would either be ignored or the trial would be a promotional trial, an excuse for getting the drug better known.

Thomas Morson Ltd, a subsidiary of Merck, Sharp and Dohme, marketed Osmosin, capsules of indomethacin that would leak out through a pinhole when osmotic pressure expanded the contents. A two centre trial was organised and involved endoscopy to detect lesions in the stomach. At one centre the work was completed quickly and showed that Osmosin was unsafe. But because the other testing centre had not completed its part of the study the company continued to promote the product until the numbers of patients suffering harm forced it to withdraw.

The bigger the attempted deception the more painful the exposure, especially in the United States, where the Opren disaster brought law suits.

The common mode of action of NSAIDs was as inhibitors of cyclo-oxygenase, the enzyme that produced the biologically active lipids called prostaglandins. Some prostaglandins had important roles in protecting the lining of the stomach from digesting itself, in maintaining urine flow and in facilitating aggregation of platelets to stem bleeding at sites of injury. Other prostaglandins caused the pain and swelling of inflammation and interfered with temperature control to cause fever. At first it was thought that there was only one cyclo-oxygenase. However, in the last decade research led by Sir John Vane and others (reviewed by Vane and Botting, 1997) has shown that there were two, named COX-1 and COX-2 with separate activities. COX-1 was normally present and generated prostaglandins responsible for protecting the stomach and maintaining urine flow but COX-2, which generated prostaglandins that produced inflammation and fever, was only released after damage to cells. NSAIDs inhibited both enzymes, but to variable degrees. After the discovery of the separate COX-2 gene in 1991, the race was on to find a drug that only inhibited COX-2. Meloxicam and etodolac were promoted as having a favourable ratio of COX-2 to COX-1 inhibition and a new COX-2 inhibitor (rofecoxib, Merck) did not cause gastrointestinal bleeding when compared to ibufrofen in healthy volunteers (Huston, 1998). Monsanto introduced a similar drug (celecoxib) and other companies were expected to follow with their own preparations. Inevitably these drugs will have adverse effects for some patients but the full spectrum of such effects will not be clear until there has been much more experience of their use.

In time there was disillusion with the NSAIDs because of concerns about gastrointestinal bleeding. In 1982 a spot check in the Royal National Hospital for Rheumatic Diseases in Bath found that the commonest drug being taken by rheumatoid arthritis patients on entry to hospital was paracetamol, either alone or compounded with another mild analgesic as in co-proxamol or benorylate.

The testing of new NSAIDS and other drugs for rheumatoid arthritis had become an industry by the 1970s. They were a source of income for the research departments of rheumatism units, often a ‘Robin Hood’ activity that helped to pay for non-drug-related research.

A company offering a new drug for clinical trial had first to submit all its data to the Dunlop Committee on the Safety of Medicines (later the Medicines Commission) to show that possible long term and short term toxicity had been sought in a variety of experimental animals and that the pharmacodynamics of the drug had been studied in normal volunteers. These requirements were considerably tightened

after the disaster that followed the introduction of the sedative drug thalidomide by the German company Chemie-Grünenthal in 1959 and sold in the UK under the name Distaval. Taken by a woman at a certain stage of pregnancy it caused phocomelia, the baby being born without proper limbs. It could also cause a particularly unpleasant form of peripheral neuritis.

At hospital level statutory local Ethics Committees were set up that also had to give their approval for a trial of a new drug. These barriers put up the cost to the company of any candidate drug. There was a sense that the patients in the trials, who were non-contracted but essential third parties, benefited in that they were always the most carefully and frequently observed patients in the hospital. They could also benefit directly by being the first to receive a more effective drug, or if on placebo, by not being exposed to unexpected toxicity. There were those who muttered about patients being turned into 'guinea-pigs'. In fact the controlled clinical trial was more effective in getting at the truth about a drug. This was illustrated by comparing the introduction of indomethacin in 1962. The real guinea pigs were the 2000 patients had been given the drug in the United States in an open trial, some of whom experienced serious gastro-intestinal complaints but there was no way of being sure that those complaints were related to the drug. Placebo controlled trials in much smaller numbers of patients in the UK produced the same proportion of adverse effects with fewer people exposed to those effects together with the certainty that those effects were drug-related.

Corticosteroids and the rheumatic diseases.

The introduction in 1948 of cortisone by Hench and Kendall in the Mayo Clinic and by Reichstein in Switzerland was followed by high expectations in the UK and a tidal wave of enthusiasm for the hormones. Importation without a licence was banned because it was feared that massive purchases by the public would cause a serious dent in the balance of payments at a time when the country was still recovering from the war. Adrenocorticotrophic hormone (ACTH) had been introduced by Thorne at the Peter Bent Brigham hospital in Boston and had been used for rheumatoid arthritis prior to Hench's announcement. It was anti-inflammatory by stimulating the patient's own suprarenal cortices to produce cortisol. It had the disadvantage of stimulating the release of mineralocorticoids, leading to fluid retention and increased blood pressure, and was prone to cause skin pigmentation because of contaminating melanocyte-stimulating hormone.

The ban on unlicenced importing of cortisone and the introduction of the National Health Service combined to provide an opportunity after 1949 to use the statistically controlled trial method to assess the long-term effects of corticosteroids and ACTH in the rheumatic diseases. While supplies were short and could only be imported with a Customs' permit, two seminal controlled trials of cortisone in the rheumatic diseases were set up, advised by Professor Austin Bradford-Hill, and his co-worker at the London School of Hygiene, Dr John Knoweldon.

Large multi-centre studies were mounted for rheumatoid arthritis and rheumatic fever with support from the Medical Research Council, The Nuffield Foundation, the Empire Rheumatism Council and a generous gift of cortisone from Merck. In those long-term studies cortisone was no better than aspirin. That those trials were largely negative did not deter many doctors from using cortisone for its dramatic short-term effects. Cortisone was addictive as the disease inevitably flared when it was withdrawn. Dr Jaques Forestier from Aix-les Bains, in a letter to the medical press, used the words "Steroid Servitude' to describe the state such sufferers were in.

One could not even claim that cortisone-type drugs did not influence the natural history of rheumatoid arthritis. They did, and for the worse. Post-corticosteroid adrenocortical suppression began to be observed. Those taking a corticosteroid were in danger of collapse from hypoadrenalism if their treatment were suddenly withdrawn or if they were subjected to the stress of an operation, accident or intercurrent pneumonia. Late complications of excessive or prolonged corticosteroid treatment began to provide new clinical signs. The thin, fragile, easy bruising skin of the shins of patients would show typical prednisolone purpura. Sometimes there were puzzling 'new moon' shaped cuts on the legs of patients caused by the sharply starched cuffs that more senior nurses wore as part of their uniform. An adhesive plaster put on such skin might pull the epidermis off when removed, much as adhesive tape on a painted wall would pull off the paint when removed. The once classical end result of the neglected rheumatoid arthritis patient, multiple contractures in the 'bed' position, (Fig 1.1) was replaced by equally crippling hypermobility and lateral instability of knees and ankles. Bones became osteoporotic, collapse fractures of the spine were increasingly frequent and were even observed in children taking corticosteroids. Limb bone fractures following minimal trauma were observed. When occurring in or near the wrist, hip or ankle they could easily be confused with a local exacerbation of the arthritis.

Hench had invented the phrase 'side effects' of corticosteroids that lulled one into thinking these were inevitable and somehow acceptable. It would have been better to use 'adverse effects'. This would have shown them in their true colours, detrimental to the patient. He also initiated the practice of commencing corticosteroid treatment with a bang, a large dose right at the start and tailing off later until symptoms returned, then raising the maintenance dose to a slightly higher level. This tended to subject the patient to alternate hope and depression as pains returned. It was kinder to 'Go low. Go slow', (a phrase that came in with penicillamine), gradually working up until there was acceptable symptom relief. This was usually at a lower dosage than the other approach.

Cortisone itself was soon followed by chemical derivatives with slightly differing spectra of activities. Prednisolone after 1955 became the standard preparation against which others were judged. It was five times stronger than cortisone. The fluorine-containing preparations dexamethasone and triamcinolone did not cause the patient to gain weight but did lead to generalised muscle wasting recognised as a steroid myopathy. Overprescription of corticosteroids by the ignorant was all too common.

Corticosteroids came into use in the 1950s for the treatment of polymyalgia rheumatica and temporal arteritis. There was no safe substitute. As with rheumatoid arthritis there was a tendency to overdose. Experience showed that the effective maintenance dose in polymyalgia might be very small; sometimes as little as 3mg a day of prednisolone was sufficient.

History will probably judge that rheumatoid arthritis patients benefited most from corticosteroid preparations designed for intra-articular use. These were presented as suspensions of poorly soluble esters in microcrystalline form that when injected into a joint were retained there, perhaps for months, giving sustained but local relief from pain and inflammation. The systemic effects were far less than with oral treatment. By the 1970s it was accepted almost everywhere that patients with arthritis were better kept up and about and as physically active as possible. One or two inflamed joints that prevented this could be treated by local injection to allow the patient to co-operate with active physiotherapy. In the Spa hospitals there was a striking reduction in the average duration of in-patient stay, (from six weeks to 14 days), and an increase in the numbers admitted accompanied this. Techniques were developed for the injection of all the main joints in the body.

Second line or Disease Modifying Antirheumatic Drugs (DMARDs).

These have also gone through phases of popularity. Gold compounds were introduced by Jaques Forestier in Aix-les Bains in 1928. Gold was used before then for tuberculosis, copying the use by Semmelweis of an arsenic compound, Salvarsan, in syphilis. Some thought that rheumatoid arthritis might be a form of tuberculous arthritis. Whatever the rationalisation, when gold was used in rheumatoid arthritis the disease usually remitted. In 1938 Philip Ellman and John Lawrence published a comparative trial of gold versus placebo. Of 20 control patients 5 improved. Of 40 treated patients 22 improved. Of the various gold compounds devised, intramuscularly injected Myocrisin, sodium aurothiomalate, was still available in 1999. An advantage of an injection as opposed to a tablet was that someone had to give it, ensuring that the patient was visited and not forgotten. By 1978 an oral gold preparation, auranofin, was prescribable but not as effective.

Serendipity marked the introduction of antimalarial drugs as DMARDs. Mepacrine was then the standard prophylaxis for travellers to countries where malaria was endemic. One such traveller had lupus and noted a remission when on mepacrine. Later mepacrine's chemical cousins, chloroquine and hydroxychloroquin were tested in rheumatoid arthritis in controlled trials at Manchester (Popert and colleagues, 1961) and at Hammersmith, (Hamilton and Scott, 1962) and shown to be effective. They differed from the other DMARD's in that they were also useful in systemic lupus and dermatomyositis. These drugs accumulated in collagen tissues, including in the lens of the eye, which could be shown to fluoresce in ultraviolet light. This did not matter so much as the occasional chloroquine damage to the fovea that had been observed in the USA. For years all patients on hydroxychloroquin were referred annually to an ophthalmologist for checking for retinal damage. In this country the use of smaller doses and with less exposure to the photochemical effects of ultraviolet light such damage was exceedingly rare. Routine expert eye checks were eventually discontinued.

Sulfasalazine came back in fashion as an effective and relatively inexpensive DMARD. Originally developed by Dr Nana Swartz in Sweden in the 1930s for the treatment of rheumatoid arthritis, it was out of vogue for that disease for 40 years. Nevertheless it continued to be available because of its effectiveness in ulcerative colitis. In the late 1970s it was re-investigated by Brian McConkey at Birmingham but was still generally ignored until championed by Howard Bird in Harrogate. It contained salicylate and sulphapyridine joined by an azo bond, but separated rapidly into its constituent parts when taken into the body. How any of the DMARDs worked was unclear.

Penicillamine was a product of the acid hydrolysis of penicillin. It had chelating activity, which inspired Walsh in 1953 to use it to promote the excretion of copper in Wilson's Disease for which it became the standard treatment. Thus there were already ten years of experience of using it in man when Dr Isadore Jaffe in the USA reasoned that penicillamine would break down the macromolecules of rheumatoid factor. He treated his patients with it and they improved.

In the UK Dr Hugh Lyle of Dista Ltd. organised an exemplary multicentre controlled trial of penicillamine in rheumatoid arthritis which confirmed Jaffe's work. Penicillamine began to supplant gold as a second line or disease modulating antirheumatic drug (DMARD). Effectiveness, adverse reactions and precautions were much the same as with gold with the interesting addition of dysgeusia, or abnormality of taste making food taste unpleasant, thought to be related to chelation of body zinc. To guard against adverse effects, the patients had to be carefully supervised and regular urine and blood tests taken. The 5-year controlled trial of DMARDs referred to on page75 showed that penicillamine was the best tolerated.

Asked how he viewed the treatment of rheumatoid arthritis over the last 40 years Dr JT Scott in retirement considered that he could manage these patients just as well with what was available then, namely aspirin and gold preparations, as with the galaxy of alternatives on the market in 1998.

Cytotoxic and immunosuppressive drugs.

The biggest advance in the treatment of more severe rheumatoid arthritis and of lupus with visceral involvement was the use of the cytotoxic anti-cancer drugs. These suppressed aggressive immune cell proliferation. Methotrexate was being tried in psoriatic arthropathy by Watson Buchanan of Glasgow when on a fellowship at Bethesda in 1962, but in most peoples' hands methotrexate caused unfavourable changes in the indices of liver function. It went out of favour until it was realised that only low doses of the order of 10 mg once a week were needed. (Hughes, 1994).

Azathioprine was the best corticosteroid-sparing immunosuppressive, but 'When you needed a miracle, and only a miracle would do' cyclophosphamide became the drug of choice.

For very severe disease complicated by vasculitis, a 'bolus' dose of cyclophosphamide, up to 500 mg intravenously, cushioned by a large and simultaneous intravenous dose of methylprednisolone came to be used and could be life saving. Cyclosporin was introduced in transplantation medicine for the prevention of immune rejection of organ replacement. Its use as monotherapy in rheumatoid arthritis to suppress auto-immune disease was at first of doubtful success and there were problems with renal toxicity. However with more experience it was finding a place in the treatment of psoriatic arthropathy as an adjunct to methotrexate. The combination was also used in vasculitis complicating rheumatoid arthritis and systemic lupus. There were hopes that its very early use in rheumatoid arthritis would prevent the disease from becoming chronic.

Future hopes for the cure of rheumatoid arthritis centred on the cytokines. At the Kennedy Institute Dr Mark Feldman predicted that Tumour Necrosis Factor-antibody (TNFα-AB) would stop inflammatory arthritis. Professor R Maini, Director of the Institute, obtained a supply of the antibody from Centecor, a biomedical company. He showed that it could bring about a temporary remission of rheumatoid arthritis in about 70% of those treated with it, thus opening up a new experimental approach to the treatment of the disease. Prof George Nuki noted that the injection of a protein material was liable to induce toxic shock. A report in the '*Lancet*' (Ault, 1999) suggested that TNFα-AB therapy might increase the liability of rheumatoid arthritis sufferers to secondary infections. There were, however, many other ways in which the activity of TNFα- might be modified and this became an area of intense research.

Research interest has also shifted to the study of phosphodiesterase enzymes, subtypes of which are involved in the production of chronic inflammation. Selective inhibitors of these are being developed for possible use in rheumatoid arthritis A more radical yet successful approach was immune ablation with subsequent stem cell rescue (Durez et. al, 1998).

Treatment of ankylosing spondylitis.

The half-century has seen a vast improvement in the management of ankylosing spondylitis. In the1960's and 70's the average interval between the onset of symptoms and correct diagnosis was seven years. Many young men and women suffered for years diagnosed as 'slipped disc'. With the establishment of the National Ankylosing Spndylitis Society recognition of the disease by doctors was sharpened

In 1939 radiotherapy to the spine or hips was used to relieve symptoms and improve mobility. This was an advance on the disastrous treatment in plaster beds or rigid corsets still advocated in some of the French literature up until 1964. Phenylbutazone supplanted radiotherapy for pain relief from 1950 onwards. Kellgren taught that ankylosing spondylitis subjects not only felt better with exercise but that their sedimentation rates improved. But to exercise when in pain required considerable motivation and motivation could not be prescribed like a pill. Accordingly in 1972 patients were admitted to the Royal National Hospital for Rheumatic Diseases in Bath in groups of 10 or more and given progressive group exercises over a period of three weeks. Measurements were taken and patients were readmitted in one year. They were fitter and more of them able to keep at work.

Out of this arose the National Ankylosing Spondylitis Society whose members formed branches that made arrangements with local hospitals to continue programmes supervised by physiotherapists. Physiotherapists responded to the challenge and took an active part in spreading and developing the message countrywide. Today it is rare today to see younger sufferers who have become bent up like a question mark. There was little evidence to show that the stiffening process itself was inhibited, but a patient whose spine stiffened in the erect posture was not handicapped from most daily activities unless the hips were involved and for them total hip replacement arthroplasty was available.

The treatment of gout.

Gout is the clinical expression of a supersaturated solution of sodium biurate in the plasma. Supersaturated solutions form easily but may precipitate sodium biurate as microcrystals. Such crystals can start an acute inflammatory reaction (acute gout) or accumulate more or less painlessly to form chalky deposits (gouty tophi). The traditional treatment of the acute gouty attack with colchicine gave way after 1949 to phenylbutazone and later to indomethacin. The latter had a dramatic effect on the painful inflammation but little effect on urate blood levels.

Along with urea and creatinine, uric acid is one of the three main pathways of nitrogen excretion and excess is normally got rid of through the urine, hence its name. There are many contributory causes of gout, classed either as over production or under excretion of uric acid.

Serendipity contributed to the conquest of gout. Probenecid and sulphinpyrazone were drugs designed in the early 1950s to affect the renal tubules so as to reduce the loss of penicillin in the urine when this antibiotic was in short supply. It was noticed that they also increased renal uric acid excretion. They were effective in curing gout except in those patients who had already acquired gouty renal damage.

The treatment of choice became allopurinol, introduced in 1958, a drug originally designed to conserve the anti-folic acid drug 6-mercaptopurine in cancer therapy. This inhibited the enzyme xanthine oxidase and thus the last stages of urate production. Allopurinol was outstandingly safe and its continued use not only normalised the serum level of urate but allowed existing urate deposits to dissolve back into the blood stream and be excreted.

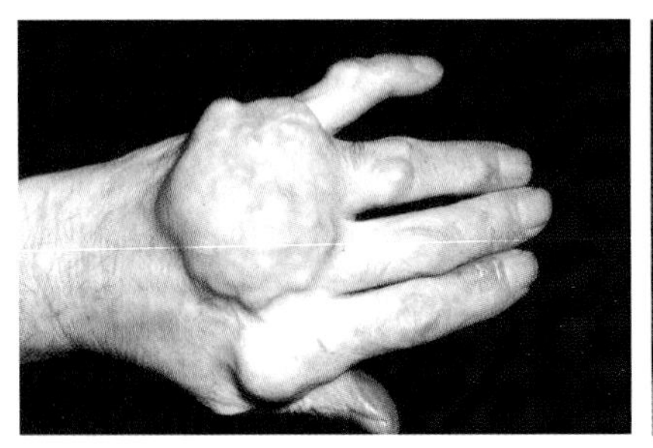

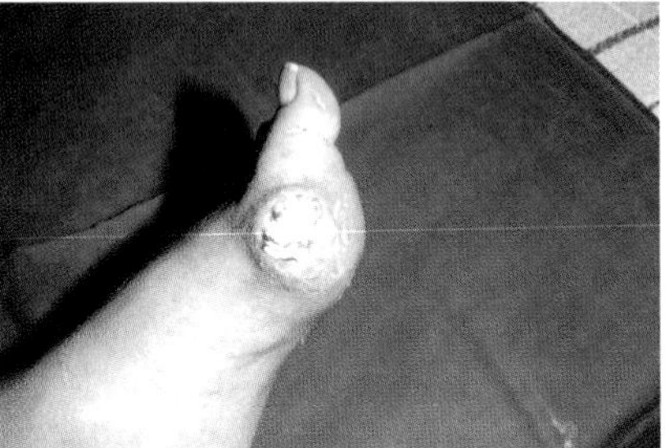

Fig 12.1. Tophacious gout on hand and toe.

Fig 12.1 shows an example of tophaceous gout as it used to be seen. After the introduction of allopurinol any patient who had gout was either not getting proper advice or not following it.

Drug treatment of osteoarthritis.

Osteoarthritis becomes more common with age, as judged by radiological or postmortem studies, yet most of it is painless and does not seriously curtail mobility. It is only serioiusly disabling or very painful when it is severe or precocious. Then the treatment is surgical.

But for lesser degrees of severity the NSAIDs provide some relief. The truth is that drugs for the condition have changed little since 1948.

There have been a succession of attempts to treat osteoarthritis by artificially lubricating the joint. It seemed to be the logical thing to do when findings at operation or autopsy showed obvious signs of wear. These included abrasion with loss of the layer of articulating cartilage, exposure and polishing of the underlying bone, and in the knee, ridging and grooving of the articulating surface in the plane of rotation of one bone on the other. Loss of lubrication was made clinically plausible because the patient might complain of stiffness of movement. In the hip high friction damage to the surface of the joint could often be heard (and felt) as a grating noise as the patient took weight on the joint and attempted to walk. Occasionally this was so marked as to give a good imitation of the 'cog-wheel' rigidity of Parkinson's disease.

The first attempts directly to improve lubrication in osteoarthritis involved putting oil in the joint. GD Kersley recalled that commercial proprietary 'Three-in-One' oil was once tried. It did not work, of course, because oil like any foreign substance was rapidly scavenged from the joint by the phagocytic action of the synovial lining. Unsuccessful attempts were made at Edinburgh and South Middlesburgh to devise an artificial water miscible lubricant that would abide in the cavity of the joint. Other materials tested included chondroitin sulphuric acid, the viscous polysaccharide derived from cartilage, and more recently solutions of the sodium salt of hyaluronic acid, the naturally occurring mucinous substance in synovial fluid.

Huskisson and Donnelly found sodium hyaluronate ('Hyalgin') to be superior to placebo when injected into knees with mild to moderate osteoarthritis. They reviewed the literature and concluded that it was a useful addition to the treatment of this condition. They speculated about the mode of action but did not think that this related only to the lubricating properties of the preparation.

The Treatment of Osteoporosis and Osteomalacia

Compared to French colleagues UK rheumatologists have only relatively recently brought bone diseases centre stage to their scene.

In an iliac crest bone biopsy osteomalacia shows as widened osteoid seams while in osteoporosis the bone trabeculae are thin and disconnected. Osteomalacia is either of alimentary origin (dietary depletion or malabsorption) or caused by abnormalities of Vitamin D (calciferol) processing in liver and kidney. All causes of osteomalacia have become treatable. It was not always so. The chemical structure of Vitamin D was worked out in the early 1920's along with the realisation that ultraviolet radiation was needed to turn vegetable and animal provitamins into calciferol. Calciferol cured most causes of osteomalacia and rickets. Fifty years later it was shown that calciferol was changed to calcitriol, the active end product, by hydroxylation in the liver and kidneys. When calcitriol or its equivalent, alphacalcidol, became available 'Vitamin-D resistant rickets' became treatable.

The tendency to osteoporosis in all persons increased with age in both sexes but was additionally contributed to by factors susceptible to treatment. These were immobilisation, systemic illnesses, smoking, poor diet and low levels of gonadal hormones. In the elderly the distinction of osteoporosis from other bone diseases was often blurred. Many also had low blood levels of vitamin D that in turn stimulated parathyroid over-activity.

In the 1940's Fuller Albright in Boston had drawn attention to osteoporosis and noted the connection with depletion of oestrogen at the menopause. By 1955 the Medical Research Council had set up a Unit in Leeds under the direction of Dr Chris Nordin to research into osteoporosis. He established ways of quantifying osteoporosis. In1961, having shown that osteoporotic subjects habitually took less calcium in their diets than normal subjects, he suggested that a long period of calcium deficiency could permanently tilt the balance of bone formation and destruction towards bone loss. A daily intake of calcium 1 g per day, taken indefinitely, was recommended. The next landmark in the treatment of osteoporosis was the work of Lindsay, Hart, Aitken and colleagues (1976) in Glasgow. They studied women who had had their ovaries removed so as to ensure a known date for loss of ovarian function. They followed the bone morphology and fracture rates in their patients for twenty years. Compared with controls, those on an oestrogen (mestranol) lost less cortical bone and had fewer fractures than those on placebo. Numerous studies of hormone replacement therapy (HRT) in postmenopausal women confirmed their findings. By 1990 there was evidence for other benefits from HRT including a sharp drop in deaths from coronary heart disease and stroke, a reduced risk of Alzheimer's disease and less tooth loss from peri-odontitis. There was evidence of increased quality and duration of life. But studies after ten years of HRT indicated an increase in the ascertainment of, but not necessarily deaths from, breast cancer, partly explained by saving women from fatal heart disease. In 1961 sodium fluoride had been introduced for the treatment of osteoporosis. It reliably increased trabecular bone density but not bone strength. Liablity to limb bone fracture was if anything increased and fluoride treatment was abandoned.

Calcitonins were used from about 1975 first as injections later by nasal inhalation. They inhibited osteoclasts, the cells that break down bone, and thus decreased age-related loss of bone density. The cost was high and the effect meagre. An important milestone in the fight against osteoporosis in the UK was the founding of the National Osteoporosis Society in 1986. At that time there were practitioners who said they had never seen osteoporosis. They had, of course, but diagnosed it as fractures and did not make the connection with the underlying bone weakness. The Society's strategy was first to make women aware of the problem, exemplified by the exponential rise in potentially fatal hip fractures. The public, worried about their aunts and mothers, went to their family doctors. They in turn passed the problem on to the hospital specialists. The public also turned to the politicians to 'do something'. In time the politicians took notice.

The subsequent global rise of awareness of osteoporosis caused drug companies to perceive a market and they responded with research. One result was another class of osteoclast inhibitors, the bisphosphonates. These were developed from water-softening agents used by the detergents industry. One of them, etidronate, given cyclically with calcium, reduced the incidence of spinal fractures. A whole family of more powerful bisphosphonates followed. Ibandronate, one of the most recent, needed only to be given intravenously once every three months. Bisphosphonates did not have the benefits of HRT with respect to the cardiovascular system.

In 1995 selective oestrogen receptor modulators (SERMS) were introduced. They were analogues of tamoxifen, long used to inhibit breast cancers and known to protect women against osteoporosis. One of these, raloxifene, blocked receptors for oestrogen in the breast and uterus but acted as a pro-oestrogen for receptors in the bones and cardiovascular system. In 1997 raloxifene was approved by the Food and Drug Administration in the USA for the prevention of osteoporosis in postmenopausal women.

Meunier's group in 1992 reported from France a successful intervention to protect elderly institutionalised women against low bone density and fractures. They had given the women vitamin D and calcium supplements over three years. Compared with controls, the treated women had fewer fractures. The method has since been used in 'free-living' elderly men and women.

New and more selective drugs for osteoporosis are likely to be discovered following the elucidation of the factors that determine the differentiation of of osteoclasts (bone destroying cells) from haematopoetic precursors. This has made it possible to produce unlimited numbers of osteoclasts *in vitro*. Previously available treatments that tended to block both osteoblasts (bone forming cells) as well as osteoclasts could slow or halt the osteoporotic process but could do little to build new bone. Selective osteoclast inhibitors can now be sought more easily.

Chapter 13
Complementary Rheumatology, Alternative Rheumatology and the Misrepresentation of Drugs and Devices.

The aches and pains lumped together as rheumatism have always attracted unorthodox practitioners and suppliers of cures. They range from sincere well-intentioned healers to the commercial vendors of useless and sometimes dangerous drugs and devices.

Complementary Medicine

Temporary pain and discomfort and subsequent improvement through healing is the natural history of nearly all episodes of back pain, yet operations for back pain were four times as common in the United States as in the UK for no good reason. Newer methods of imaging the spines of normal subjects had revealed that degeneration and prolapses of intervertebral discs taken as indications for surgery were common in persons who were completely pain-free (Deyo, 1998). The implication was that most patients operated on would have been wiser to have waited until symptoms improved. It was in the area of back pain, with its high natural recovery rate, that most practitioners of complementary medicine tended to operate.

Professor E Ernst of Exeter University preferred the word 'complementary' to 'alternative' medicine since most people, and this included over 60% of those with rheumatic problems, used both mainline medicine as well as complementary medicine. Complementary medicine had royal approval. On October 22nd 1997 the Prince of Wales called for more co-operation between the National Health Service and complementary practitioners . In 1999 he arranged informal meetings of the two sides at his Highgrove House.

A cynical view would be that consulting complementary medicine relieved the burden on doctors by 'treating' patients with trivial or self-limiting complaints while they got better, when medical inaction might have been construed as neglect. Others considered 'there might be something in it' or 'live and let live'.

Complementary medicine has been urged to prove its case by scientifically designed clinical trials.

A British Broadcasting Corporation programme (June 9th 1998) surveyed 45,000 people and found that one in four used complementary medicine. Adrian White was the presenter and acupuncturist. White used stainless steel needles. 'It frees energy lines or meridians.' 'Not pricking because of the lines, but just to give the energy lines a boost' He took the view that 'on balance *(it was)* a true effect in back pain, but for osteoarthritis the evidence is mixed'. He had never seen any evidence that meridians actually existed and suggested a counter-irritant mechanism.

The history of manipulation and bone setting goes back millennia. Very little has changed except that methods and designations have multiplied and a few have achieved official recognition in some countries. Orthodox Medicine has never sufficiently recognised the perceived value to a person in pain of the laying on of friendly hands, whether it be stroking or the touch of skin on skin from a physiotherapist, a manipulator or the doctor doing a careful physical examination.

Of the heterodox or 'Fringe Medicine' methods of treatment, as Brian Inglis (1964) called them, it is chiropractic that is the most likely to be acceptable to orthodox medicine, together with those sects of osteopathy which have moved nearer to orthodox medical training. (Some have begun to replace primary care doctors in parts of the United States where most of the doctors try to become specialists). Chiropractors take X-rays and have some chance of knowing rather than imagining what is happening under the skin to their patients. Nevertheless a survey by Ernst and Assendelft in a *British Medical Journal* editorial concluded that 'On the basis of current evidence, it seems uncertain whether chiropractic does more good than harm'.

All types of complementary practitioners, chiropractors, osteopaths, acupuncturists, homeopaths, aroma therapists and herbalists give systematised explanations of what they do and why, which is comforting to patients even if the explanations are not evidence-based. It is for back pain with its high natural remission rates that most have satisfactory consultations with complementary therapists.

The Drug Hucksters

Most industrialised countries have legislated against false and misleading claims for treatments for defined diseases such as cancer or rheumatoid arthritis. The word 'rheumatism', however, is not definable in scientific terms and there are no penalties for false claims to cure it. The Arthritis and Rheumatism Council has dropped the word 'Rheumatism' and changed its name to Arthritis Research Campaign. Same charity, same initials.

Chronic rheumatic disease sufferers have always been the targets of hyped-up promotions of ineffective or bogus remedies. In the USA the money they spent on such products in the 1950's was more than that spent on orthodox medicines. This prompted an American study (Walrad, 1960) entitled 'The Misrepresentation of Arthritis Drugs and Devices' (Figure 13.1) that attempted to combat the enormous trade in unproven remedies. It was based on an analysis of 909 questionnaires returned by arthritis sufferers[12] who were asked if they had ever bought a product advertised as being a cure for arthritis. 129 such products were reported. Only ten people considered that they had been cured.

The survey also listed 944 other arthritis treatments of which the respondents were aware. These included drugs, vitamin products, food supplements, herbal preparations, liniments, devices and books advising on diets and lifestyle changes. The drugs and other preparations were heard about through the media, particularly television. The devices, which outnumbered the drugs and liniments, included massage machines, vibrators, heat pads, magnetic belts, special corsets and the like. They were mostly bought through drug stores. The misleading books included Dan Dale Alexander's '*Arthritis and Common Sense*' and Bernard Aschner's '*Arthritis can be cured*', that had been sold in their millions.

12 Approximately 2/3rds rheumatoid arthritis and 1/3rd osteoarthritis.

ARTHRITIS DRUGS AND DEVICES IN THE UNITED STATES

A REPORT

to

Committee on Arthritis Advertising

The Arthritis and Rheumatism Foundation

by

Ruth Walrad

Research Consultant

Copyright, 1960
by the
Arthritis and Rheumatism Foundation
New York, New York

Fig. 13.1

There has been no similar survey of misleading arthritis drugs and devices in the United Kingdom. A publication entitled 'Health Watch' under the chairmanship of Prof. John Garrow of Northwick Park Hospital attempted to guide its readership as to the validity of claims for treatments in general. Its former editor, Caroline Richmond, wrote: 'I would like to do a study of alternative rheumatism remedies, which I'm sure is the biggest of all the bogus health industries. I know that even conspicuous sceptics get the most awful remedies foisted on them by their middle-class friends (working class people seem to be more sensible)'.

Most lay people who suffer from what they consider to be 'rheumatism' do not have arthritis (inflammation of the joints). Few would know that there are over a hundred different rheumatic diseases for only some of which there are specific treatments and expectations of cure. Rheumatologists recognise the 'inevitable seventy per cent' of sufferers from *any* rheumatic disease who consider themselves briefly improved or even cured by *any* treatment. Truly active treatments have to do better than that. Placebo treatment can sometimes be followed by both clinical and biological improvement, as was shown in Chapter 2, figure 2.5. Even sufferers from severe osteoarthritis of the hip will consider themselves improved on injections of dilute salt solution, as has been shown in the placebo arms of placebo-controlled clinical trials of candidate treatments. In such circumstances it is easy for the drug hucksters to push inappropriate remedies at high prices and acquire testimonials and even a public following.

Sometimes the contents of a cure are not as advertised. A product sold as a Chinese herbal medicine for rheumatism was found to be fortified with cortisone, others had high lead levels or contained substances that might cause abnormal heart rhythms or impotence, despite being labelled 'all natural'. This has prompted calls for herbal products to be registered and controlled for safety, content and efficacy in the same way as ordinary medicines.

A typical scam was 'Seatone', the dried and powdered gonads of the Pacific green-lipped mussel farmed in the Marlborough Sounds of New Zealand. Although classified as a food supplement, it was presented as tablets and backed by some pseudoscience. It achieved a world-wide sale as a cure for rheumatoid arthritis until controlled trials at St Bartholomew's Hospital (Dr E. Huskisson) showed it to be indistinguishable from dried fishmeal. It made a substantial contribution, in its day, to the New Zealand balance of payments.

The Internet provided a new and un-policed medium for promoting bogus remedies. A brief visit to some of the sites disclosed extraordinary claims. The price of the product was usually in proportion to the hype. Copper bracelets containing five pennyworth of copper sell for five pounds. One can buy 'Magnetic ear clips' to be attached to the ear at so-called meridian points as a new form of acupuncture. Or one can rub on WONDERGEL advertised as preserving the rain forests. (For no logical reason. The main ingredients were the usual counter-irritants, methylsalicylate, menthol and eucalyptus oil with *Aloe Vera* mucilage and other thickening agents). Herbal remedies such as alfalfa, burdock root *(Arctium),* wormwood *(Artemisia)* and comfrey *(Symphytum),* long debunked and some the subject to United States 'cease and desist' orders, were touted on the Internet along with undefined products such as Dragon Oil. They were described as 'good for' or 'aiding the healing of" arthritis. The word cure was usually avoided, presumably for legal reasons.

Chapter14
A Patient's Story

This history is of rheumatology and of rheumatologists, their efforts to help their patients and to unravel the secrets of the rheumatic diseases with the hope of providing prevention and cure. But what was it like to be a patient, finding that making one's way in the world was obstructed by an unknown enemy inside? Doctors are probably better doctors if they can view their patient's problems objectively. But it is sometimes impossible not to feel involved while seeing the courage and optimism with which some face their problems.

In today's jargon, rheumatologists are 'providers' and patients are 'purchasers'. It is time to hear from one of the purchasers, one who has been affected by one of the more severe forms of rheumatoid arthritis.

"I was born in October 1924 so when the war broke out I was just 15. I was called up in 1941 and trained as part of a bomber crew and was shot down over Cologne and served the rest of the war in a prisoner of war camp in East Germany. I escaped from East Berlin after being taken prisoner by the Russians and made my way (with some difficulty) back to the UK. After the war I went into advertising and selling, selling edible oils and fats for Unilever. And chocolates for Fuller's in Hammersmith. I switched from selling chocolates to selling stone when in 1960 I joined a quarrying firm as Sales Manager. That was quite a jump for someone who up to then had thought 'scalpings' was a disease!

It was in 1965 that I first noticed some swelling of my fingers and not feeling well. Both my GP and the hospital consultant thought at first it was because of my lifestyle and that I had been doing too much, but later they showed me the result of a Rose test for rheumatoid arthritis which had come back strongly positive. I was put on gold injections, three or four courses.

By the second course it worked wonders and I could go back to playing golf. After more gold I had the usual tests on my blood and urine. Then the GP decided he would not give me any more, apparently he was frightened of side effects.

I went to a naturopath who told me to fast for 10 to 14 days- it worked for a while but you can't go on fasting forever.

I got worse and was back in hospital for a two and a half months. I used to 'escape' at night secretly to visit a friend. One night my joints were so painful I couldn't get back. I practically had to be carried back and it was then the Registrar first put me on steroids. I remember seeing a card at that time which said I had SLE cells and I thought this was the end of me. But they reassured me that this sometimes happened in rheumatoid arthritis.

About 1970 I bought my own quarrying business. It made a lot of money which helps when you have arthritis and have to get something done.

Then I was put on penicillamine and after that a combination of Indocid and Imuran. That helped for a long time, with occasional injections in my joints if one or other of them flared up. I developed a small lump behind the nipple that they said was caused by the Imuran, -anyway, it went away.

The first surgery was on my hands. The surgeon took off a bursa, I think you call them, on the back of each hand. The second operation happened when I was 59. I got sent to a general surgeon for a lump in the left groin. When he operated he found a cyst full of fluid. I had to have a hip replacement operation in 1988. Then I got a painful neck and problems with the nerves at the top of my neck. I had an operation to fix the first and second vertebrae. After the operation I was in a coma for several days until they woke up to the fact that I had been on a small dose of steroids for a long time and they had not been giving me any. Some years after that I got 'necrotising fasciitis--the newspapers called it the' Flesh-eating bug'- and I had to have a gangrenous bit of my foot removed. It was slow to heal and it meant I could not exercise. After that I had a coronary artery bypass which healed OK but the cuts they made to get the leg veins for grafting the arteries wouldn't heal and got infected. It meant skin grafts which at first wouldn't 'take' but which eventually did.

This was followed by more weakness in my arms and legs and it was back to the neurosurgeon again to fix the third, fourth, fifth and sixth vertebrae in my neck. There were other problems. The left ankle became painful. It appears that as I had to walk on the inside of my foot there is too much strain on the lower end of the fibula. I have mild diabetes. The skin on the backs of the hands and forearms tears very easily, but it heals soon. I have to wear elastic stocking to minimise the swelling of my legs but once when I wasn't wearing them I accidentally knocked my foot and got a hole in the skin which poured out fluid before it started to bleed. My final two operations have been a replacement right knee in 1997 and a replacement ankle the following year

But there are good bits: good eyesight, good hearing, good memory, I may be falling to bits but my brain is still working.

Exercise? Yes, I set the alarm for 7 every morning and drive off to the swimming pool. I do 20 lengths non-stop."

Chapter 15

Successes and Failures and Future Trends.

In the last 50 years the *clinical successes* have been many:

- The disappearance of rheumatic fever and rheumatic heart disease.
- The cure of tuberculous and septic arthritis with antibiotics.
- The cure of gout.
- Prosthetic replacements for damaged joints, especially hips.
- The recognition and successful treatment of polymyalgia rheumatica and temporal arteritis.
- The exploration of the anti-cardiolipin syndrome and the prevention of abortion in young women with lupus.
- There have been successes in finding treatments, (but not yet cures) for osteoporosis and Paget's disease.
- The recognition and successful treatment of arthritis in Whipple's disease and Lyme disease.
- Haemophilic arthropathy is now controllable with factor 8.
- Wegener's granulomatosis and allied forms of vasculitis are now controllable.
- The various manifestations of chondrocalcinosis and calcific tendinitis have been recognised.
- The total management of juvenile chronic arthritis is also a success story. There are children, now grandparents, who but for Taplow would long ago have perished.
- The medical, physical and surgical management of rheumatoid arthritis and its complications is a success story. The duration and quality of the lives of patients have been improved and some complications, such as peripheral neuropathy, are now rare. However the effective drugs now available have often brought their own complications, such as gastrointestinal ulceration, osteoporosis and impaired immunity to infections.
- Similar considerations mark the improvement in the quality and duration of life of patients with systemic lupus.

Yet one must recognise *the clinical failures.* Despite enormous improvements in the outlook for patients, rheumatoid arthritis remains a common, single, well-defined, medical disease for which neither cause nor cure has been found. Nor have the cause and cure of ankylosing spondylitis, psoriatic arthropathy and Reiter's disease been found. We can make life much better for ankylosing spondylitis sufferers but we still cannot entirely relieve the symptoms nor prevent the chronicity of the disease. Thus of 100 patients with adult onset ankylosing spondylitis after a mean of 16 years 51.5 % of the patients were employed full time. Giving up work occurred after a mean of 15.6 years, more frequently in women and where there had been poor education, uveitis, bamboo spine and co-morbidity. After 20 years of disease more than 80% of patients complained of daily pain and stiffness and 60% took large doses of drugs. (Gran and Skomsvoll, 1997)

The manifestations of osteoarthritis have failed to find a medical cure.

Back pain remains the commonest rheumatic cause of loss of time from industry despite progress in rehabilitation first by recognising the high natural recovery rate (see Chapter 13) and secondly by the policy of early activation and mobilisation.

The scientific successes were the discovery of rheumatoid factor and the Hargrave's (lupus) cell. They alerted medicine to the auto-immune nature of these diseases. They gave objective tests for diagnosis, classification and epidemiology. Later the discovery of the association of the leucocyte antigen HLA B27 and ankylosing spondylitis was a scientific breakthrough, indicating the genetic predisposition.

In osteoarthritis Radin and his associates (1972) pointed to the trade-off between increasing bone density and decreasing resistance of weight-bearing cartilage to impact forces, an important step in our understanding of this disease. It may yet bear fruit in that wearing 'trainer' type shoes with impact-absorbing heels should reduce the burden of osteoarthritis of the hip in later years.

But it is salutary to ask how funding by the Arthritis and Rheumatism Council, the Oliver Bird Fund and other charities has over the years contributed to the beginnings of these successes?

We have seen how the ARC's response to Charnley's development of his prosthetic hip was to refuse him a grant[13]. Later its Research Committee advised Professor Hughes to discontinue his anti-cardiolipin research. It would be hard to claim that the original discoveries underlying the *clinical* successes were owed to ARC or Oliver Bird charitable money. Most successful drugs for rheumatic diseases resulted from serendipitous discoveries in other fields, often the result of unpredictable, sometimes unimaginable, coincidences. But the existence of what might be called the research industry, whether funded by commercial, state or charitable money has, however, done much to ensure the delivery of the benefits of these discoveries to those who need them.

ARC and Oliver Bird Fund donations have on the other hand contributed to some of the *scientific* successes. Examples include the discovery of HLA-DR4 as a predisposing factor for rheumatoid arthritis, the hypothesis that rheumatoid arthritis is driven by T-cells, and the exploration of anti-tumour necrosis factor- therapies.

Klemperer's concept of rheumatoid and lupus as collagen diseases caused money to be poured out, seemingly without questioning whether this was the right concept. The early results were not clinically relevant to rheumatic diseases although

13 He was, however, supported by the Nuffield Foundation.

later results did bear on the abnormalities of collagen in rare congenital diseases of bones and joints. A help with common diseases has been the characterisation of the N- and C- terminal fragments of the collagen molecule and their use as markers for osteoporosis and Paget's disease where breakdown of bone collagen is an important part of the pathological process. Could all the money have been better spent? The money has built up rheumatology research in this country at an annual cost of about £30m. Much of this is paid to support biologists, medically qualified or not, doing basic research that, they hope, will in turn develop clinical applications.

The avowed strategy of the Arthritis Research Campaign (ARC) is to ensure that there is a properly supported academic rheumatology presence in every university and teaching hospital and to endow positions where these might be otherwise lost. Thus rheumatology research is poised to expand even further in the next millenium. It is a valid criticism that research approved by a committee will favour the exploration of existing lines of research that the committee members know about. New lines of research will be looked at very carefully before being supported. A committee, like a second-hand car dealer, doesn't like to buy anything that isn't already running. Yet committees that judge research projects by peer review are now so accepted that it is difficult to see how else to proceed. Like democracy, it may not be perfect but there is no better way. That overall the system of peer review does 'work' is shown by the numerous scientific discoveries that at some stage have been given the approval of a committee.

Could evidence-based ways be found to improve committee judgements? It is said that at one time in Germany the Volkswagen Foundation used to allocate most of its funds to projects approved by a committee but kept some money to be allotted at random to applicants who had been turned down. Follow-up of what happened could have provided a basis for an audit of committee procedure.

One benefit to rheumatology of having well funded academic units in teaching hospitals has been to so raise the standing of rheumatology within the medical profession that it is attractive to good young doctors. And if 'Chance favours the prepared mind' there is always the hope that it may prepare their minds for discoveries at the bedside.

Future Trends

How will rheumatology develop in the next millennium? Leaving aside Acts of God, nuclear wars and global warming there are some indications. Rheumatology has already lost a considerable proportion of its NHS beds. In some hospitals it has become almost an outpatient speciality. This trend is likely to continue as early diagnosis and skills in using available drugs and intra-articular corticosteroids make it less important to admit patients to hospital. Currently much research is going into finding markers in early rheumatoid arthritis that can indicate a good or bad prognosis. The hope is to identify those who, untreated, would be expected to do badly and to give them treatments to prevent the progression of the disease. This can be traced back to the days of the rheumatism service at Stoke Mandeville Hospital, where Alan Hill and his colleagues noted that arthritis sufferers whose blood contained raised amounts of rheumatoid factor when first seen, or who developed raised amounts during the first year of their disease, could be expected to have a worse outcome than those who did not show this. Since the 1970's early arthritis clinics have been set up in many hospitals, particularly in Birmingham and Leeds in order to find other markers of a poor outcome and to find treatments that, if given early enough, would prevent this. As with all attempts at prevention, the question has to be asked, 'How do you know that, but for what you do, what you are trying to prevent would have happened anyway?'

It is likely that there will be increased exploration by rheumatologists of the interface with sports medicine, with muscle diseases and with pain physiology.

The 3 billion base pairs that make up the human genome will all soon be identified and mapped. Geneticists classify the inflammatory rheumatic diseases as 'multifactorial' meaning that predisposition to them will be found to be linked to a large number of different genetic influences. Mapping the human genome makes it likely that these will be discovered and enormous effort, money and technological invention has already been spent on this quest. Le Fanu, (1999) however, has suggested that this may be a false dawn. He has pointing out that a single mutation in the gene that is linked to an inherited disease (retinitis pigmentosa) can be found in an individual who does not have the disease, while another inherited disease (cystic fibrosis) can be caused by 200 or more different mutations of the the nucleotides that code for it.

The ageing of the population will emphasise osteoporosis and there will be (already are) closer links with women's health clinics. Hip fracture will become more common. Mending hip fractures will be a routine that hospitals may devolve to specialist private contractors much as some now contract out their waiting lists of varicose vein operations and cataract operations. Anti-osteoporosis therapy will be part of their routine service.

Tissue engineering is a rapidly expanding field. Already it is possible to grow articular cartilage suitable for grafting. Perhaps in the future we will be able to regenerate lost limbs or destroyed joints. In this and in other aspects of the assessment and diagnosis of rheumatic diseases the newer methods of imaging will increasingly complement and may replace traditional radiography.

In Chapter 4 Dr Hazleman, the 1999 President of the British Society for Rheumatology, was quoted in relation to the perceived bias of ARC's funding towards basic research and away from clinical research. One university (Newcastle) has appointed a non-medical Professor of Rheumatology. If there is such a bias it is likely to continue as by its nature 'near-patient' research is relatively soft science when compared with laboratory research. For 'near-patient' research to have the smaller share of a cake does not matter as long as the cake itself continues to grow in size, as there is every indication that it will.

Rheumatology has so far failed to meet the challenge of the lack of correlation between anatomical disease and pain. There will be more research into the mechanism and perception of pain. There is one other unsolved puzzle. Figure 15.1 shows the hands of a patient who had had a meningioma removed and who was left with a right hemiplegia. He subsequently developed rheumatoid arthritis. The manifestations of rheumatoid arthritis, which included swelling of joints and tendon sheaths, nodule

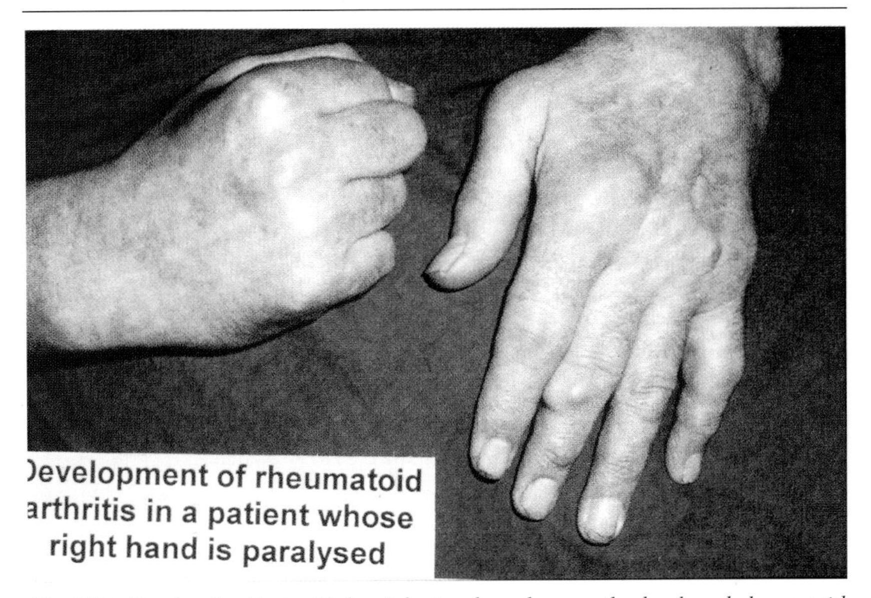

Fig 15.1. Hands of patient with hemiplegia who subsequently developed rheumatoid arthritis.

formation and ulnar deviation of the fingers were totally suppressed in the paralysed hand. The late Prof. John Ball at Manchester thought this was one of the most profound observations in the natural history of the disease. Perhaps all applicants for funds for research into rheumatoid arthritis should be questioned 'How will your plan help explain this observation?'

The AIDS virus interferes with immunity through poisoning CD4 lymphocytes. Yet AIDS often presents as a rheumatic disease that has been considered autoimmune in nature, specifically Reiter's Syndrome, Sjögren's Syndrome or psoriatic arthropathy. Does this mean that these conditions are caused by the awakening of a sleeping virus rather than by an auto-immune process? It also suggests that the pathogenesis of these conditions is different from that of rheumatoid arthritis.

There are planned changes in information technology that will affect rheumatology. The next generation of doctors and most other hospital personnel will have to be computer and keyboard literate (Table 15.1). In preparation for The Decade of the Bone and Joint, 2000-2010, the International League of Associations for Rheumatology (ILAR) has gone on line to provide the world rheumatology community with information about events and discoveries.

What will happen in the rheumatological utopia when the cure for rheumatoid arthritis is found? There will be no need for so many rheumatologists and no need for so many academic units. Those concerned will diversify into other fields. Let us hope that it will not take another half century.

Time frame for NHS information strategy

1998-2000

- Problems of millennium bug to be overcome
- NHS Direct (the patient helpline) to go nationwide
- National NHS email system to be completed
- All GP practices to be on the NHSNet
- Electronic health records start in selected GP practices

2000-2

- All appointments, radiography examinations, and laboratory requests to be booked on the NHSNet
- Community prescribing to go electronic
- Electronic library for health to be accessible on the NHSNet
- "Substantial numbers"(>35%) of hospitals to have level 3 electronic patient record systems
- First generation electronic health records to be started

2003-5

- All hospitals to have level 3 (or higher) electronic patient record system
- Transfer of electronic records among GPs possible
- Full implementation of electronic health record
- 24 hour emergency access to patient records

British Medical Journal 1998 **317** p.901

Table 15.1

References

Chapter 1

Bach F and Savage OA, 'Splenectomy in the treatment of rheumatoid arthritis, a report of three cases' *Ann Rheum Dis* (1940) **2**: pp. 47-57

Bach F, Hill NG, Preston TW and Thornton CE, 'Review of places available for rheumatic fever patients in London'. *Ann Rheum Dis* (1939) 1: pp. 210-241

Currie JP, 'Treatment of rheumatoid arthritis with Butazolidine', *Lancet* (1952) **ii**: pp. 15 - 16

Freedman A and Bach F, 'Mepacrine and rheumatoid arthritis, preliminary communication.' *Lancet* (1952) ii: p. 231

Hart FD, 'Rheumatic subcutaneous nodule formation', *Ann Rheum Dis* (1939) **1**: pp. 196-200

Kersley GD and Glyn J, 'A Concise International History of Rheumatology and Rehabilitation, Friends and Foes'. Royal Society of Medicine, London, (1991) p. 26

Moll J, 'The Heberden Society' Chapman and Hall, London, (1987), pp.143 & 303

Porritt AE and Hart FD, 'WSC Copeman, his importance in contemporary medicine' *Ann Rheum Dis* (1992) **51**: pp. 583-5

Stanworth SJ, Bhavnani M, Chattopadhya C et al., 'Treatment of Felty's syndrome with the haemopoietic growth factor granulocyte colony-stimulating factor (G-CSF)' *Quart J Med* (1998) **91:** pp. 49-56

Chapter 2

Dixon AS, Martin BK, Smith MJH, and Wood PNH, Eds., 'Salicylates, an International Symposium', J & A Churchill, London, (1963)

Duthie JJR. 'The sociological aspects of the treatment of arthritis. Notes on a visit to the USA,' *Ann Rheum Dis* (1939), **1**: pp.201-229

Kersley GD and Glyn J, 'A Concise International History of Rheumatology and Rehabilitation, Friends and Foes'. Royal Society of Medicine, (1991) p.45

Roy LMH, Alexander WRM and Duthie JJR, ' Nature of anaemia in rheumatoid arthritis. 1. Metabolism of iron.' *Ann. Rheum Dis* (1955) **14:** pp.63-72

Sinclair RJG and Duthie JJR, 'Intravenous iron in hypochromic anaemia associated with rheumatoid arthritis'. *Lancet* (1949), **2**: p.646-7

Spencer MA and Dixon AS, 'Rheumatological features of patients admitted as emergencies to acute general medical wards' *Rheum Rehab* (1981) **20**: pp. 71-3

Truelove LH and Duthie JJR, 'Effect of aspirin on the cutaneous response to the local application of an ester of nicotinic acid' *Ann Rheum Dis* (1959) **19:** pp. 137-141

Chapter 3

Beighton P, Grahame R and Bird H, 'Hypermobility of Joints', Springer Verlag, Second Edition (1983). (Third Edition in preparation)

Brewerton DA, Caffrey MFP, Hart FD et al.,'Ankylosing Spondylitis and HLA-B27' *Lancet* (1973) **1**: pp 904-907

Caffrey MFP and James DCO, 'Human lymphocyte antigen associated with ankylosing spondylitis' *Nature* (1973) **242**: p. 121

Hughes RAC, 'Hughes Syndrome: the antiphospholipid syndrome'. *J Roy Coll Phys Lond* (1998) **32**: pp. 260-4

Hamilton EBD, Williams R, Barlow KA et al., 'The arthropathy of idiopathic haemochromatosis' *Quart J Med* (1968) **37**: pp.171-82

Mathews JA and Yates DAH, 'Reduction of lumbar disc prolapse by manipulation.' *Brit Med J* (1969) **3**: pp. 696-7

Chapter 4

Andrews FM and others, the multicentre trial group, 'Penicillamine in rheumatoid arthritis' *Lancet* (1973) **I:** pp.277-280

Boyd W, 'Werner's Syndrome, (Progeria of the adult). Further pathological and biochemical observations'. *Brit Med J* (1959) **ii**: pp.920- 925

Collins DH, 'Observations on the pathology of acute rheumatism and rheumatoid arthritis.' *Ann Rheum Dis* (1939), **1**: pp.38-45

Jessop JD, O'Sullivan MM, Lewis PA et al., 'A long term 5-year randomised controlled trial of hydroxychloroquin, sodium aurothiomallate, auranofin and penicillamine in the treatment of patients with rheumatoid arthritis'. *Brit J Rheum* (1998) **37**: pp.992-1002

West HF, 'An aetiology of ankylosing spondylitis'. *Ann Rheum Dis* (1949) **8**: pp.143-148

Chapter 5

Alderson F, 'The inland resorts and spas of Britain', David and Charles. Newton Abbot, (1973)

Coates V and Delicati L, 'Rheumatoid arthritis and its treatment', H K Lewis and Co, London (1931)

Jacoby RK, Jayson MIV and Cosh JA, 'Onset, early stages, and prognosis of rheumatoid arthritis: A clinical study of 100 patients with 11-year follow-up' *Brit Med J,* (1973) **2**: pp.96-100

Thompson WAR, 'Spas that heal', A and C Black Ltd., London, (1978)

Chapter 7

Ansell BM, Personal Communication

Ansell BM, Bywaters EGL, Spencer PE, and Tyler JP, 'Looking Back 1945-1985. The Canadian Red Cross Memorial Hospital,' Published by Ansell BM, ISBN No. 0 9530992 0 2. (1997)

Arden GP, Ansell BM, Eds, 'The surgical management of juvenile chronic arthritis' Academic Press. London (1978)

Bach F, Hill NG, Preston TW and Thornton CE, 'Juvenile rheumatism in London'. *Ann Rheum Dis.* (1939) 1: p. 210-241

Bywaters EGL, Personal Communication

Bywaters EGL, Report of a three month journey to the United States on behalf of the Special Unit for Juvcnile Rheumatism at the Canadian Red Cross Memorial Hospital, Taplow. (1949) (Unpublished)

Carey R Coombs, 'Rheumatic Heart Disease' Bristol: John Wright and Sons Ltd. (1924)

Wilson MG, 'Rheumatic Fever', New York, The Commonwealth fund (1940) pp. 98-109

Woo P, Editorial. 'The growth of paediatric rheumatology' *Brit J Rheum* (1997) **36**: pp. 721-8

Chapter 8

Bradford FK and Spurling RG, (1947) 'The Intervertebral Disc' 1st edn. Thomas, Springfield, Illinois

Devas MB and Irving RE, 'The Geriatric Orthopaedic Unit,' *J Bone Jnt Surg* (Br) (1967) **48**: p. 186-7

Newman PH, 'Development of Total Hip Replacement' In Jayson M. (ed) 'Total hip replacement' (1971) Sector Publishing Ltd., London, pp. 13-25

Oliver CW, 'The role of surgery in patients with rheumatoid arthritis', *Rep Rheum Diseases* (1997) No 12

Waugh, W, 'A history of the British Orthopaedic Association. The first seventy-five years.' (1993), British Orthopaedic Association, London. p. 197

Waugh W, 'John Charnley, the Man and the Hip', (1990) Springer-Verlag, London,

Chapter 10

Bennett GA and Bauer W, 'Joint changes resulting from patella displacement and their relation to degenerative joint disease' *J Bone Jnt Surg* (1937) **19**: p. 667-682

Billings F, 'Chronic focal infections and their etiologic relations to arthritis and nephritis'. *Arch Int Med* (1912) 9: p. 484-498

Billings, F, 'Focal Infection: the Lane Medical Lectures.' New York, Appleton and Co., 1916, p. 154

Blake DR, (1998) Personal communication

Brewerton DA, Caffrey M, Hart FD et al., 'Ankylosing spondylitis and HLA-B27' *Lancet* (1973) **i**: p. 904-7

Dixon AS, Grant C, 'Acute synovial rupture, clinical and experimental observations.' *Lancet* (1965) **i**: pp.742-5

Dixon AS and Hawkins C, Eds. 'Raised Intra-articular Pressure-Clinical Consequences' (1989). The Bath Institute for Rheumatic Diseases, Bath

Hargraves MM, Richmond H and Morton R, 'Presentation of two bone marrow elements: the 'tart' cell and the 'LE' cell.' *Mayo Clin Proc.* (1948) **23**: pp. 25-28

Hutton CW, Higgs ER, Jackson PC et al., '99mTc-HMDP bone scanning in generalised nodal osteoarthritis.' *Ann Rheum Dis* (1986) **45**: 617-21 and 622-26

Kellgren JH, Moore R, 'Generalised osteoarthritis and Heberden's nodes' *Brit Med J* (1952) **i**: pp.181-87

Klemperer P, Pollack AD and Baehr G, 'Diffuse Collagen Disease- Acute disseminated lupus erythematosus and diffuse scleroderma.' *J Amer Med Ass* (1942) **119**: pp. 331-2

Panayi GS, Woolley PH and Batchelor JR, 'Genetic basis of rheumatoid disease: HLA antigens, disease manifestations, and toxic reactions to drugs.' *Brit Med J* (1978) **ii**: pp. 1326-8

Radin EL, 'Biomechanical considerations' In: 'Osteoarthritis: Diagnosis and Management', Philadelphia, W.B.Saunders (1991).Moskowitz RW, Howell WS, Goldberg VM et al., Eds

Schlosstein L, Terasaki PI, Bluestone R et al., 'High association of an HL-A antigen, W27, with ankylosing spondylitis.' *New Engl J Med* (1973) **288**: pp. 704-6

Statsny P, 'Association of the B-cell alloantigen DRw4 with rheumatoid arthritis.' *New Engl J Med* (1978) **298:** pp. 869-71

The 'Times' (May 12th 1998) report of research at the Royal National Orthopaedic Hospital under the leadership of Prof. George Bentley

Waugh W, 'A History of the British Orthopaedic Association' (1993) British Orthopaedic Association, London, p.154

Chapter 11

Vickers AJ, Rees RW and Robin A, 'Advice given by health food shops: Is it clinically safe' *J Roy Col Phys Lond.,* (1998) **32**: pp.426-7

Chapter 12

Ault B, *Lancet* (1999) **353**: p. 1770

Campion GV and Dixon AS, (1989) 'Rheumatology', Blackwell Scientific, Oxford. pp. 242-3

Dixon AS, Martin BK, Smith MJH and Wood PHN, (1963) 'Salicylates, an International

Symposium' J & A Churchill, London

Durez P, Toungouz M, Schandené L et al., 'Remission and immune reconstitution after T-cell-depleted stem-cell transplantation for rheumatoid arthritis' *Lancet,* (1998) **352**: p.881

Gross M. and Greenberg LA, (1948). 'The Salicylates- a critical bibliographic review', Millhouse Press, New Haven

Hamilton EBD and Scott JT, 'Hyroxychloroquin sulphate ('Plaquenil') in treatment of rheumatoid arthritis' *Arthr and Rheum* (1962) **5**: pp. 502-12

Hughes GRV, 'Conference reports: Methotrexate in rheumatic disease' *J Roy Col Phys Lond* (1994) **28**: p. 260

Huskisson EC and Donnelly S, 'Hyaluronic acid in the treatment of osteoarthritis of the knee' *Rheumatology* (1999) **38**: pp. 602-7

Husten l, 'Faecal blood loss avoided by Cox-2 inhibitor.' *Lancet* (1998) **352**: p. 1363

Philips, Roger, (1977) 'Wild Flowers of Britain', Pan Books, London, p. 112

Popert AJ, Meiers KAE, Sharp J et al., 'Choroquin diphosphate in rheumatoid arthritis, a controlled trial' *Ann Rheum Dis.,* (1961) **20**: pp. 18-35

Vane J, Botting J, eds. Selective COX-2 inhibitors: pharmacology, clinical effects and therapeutic potential. London: William Harvey Press, (1997): 117-25

Woolf AD & Dixon AS. 'Osteoporosis, a Clinical Guide' 2nd edition, (1998) Martin Dunitz, London

Chapter13

Deyo RA, 'Low Back Pain' *Sci Amer,* August 1998, pp. 29-33

Ernst E, 'The rise and fall of complementary medicine' *J Roy Soc Med* (1998) **91**: pp. 235-6

Ernst E and Assendelft WJJ, 'Chiropractic for low back pain' *Brit Med J* (1998) **317**: p.160

Gottlieb, S. 'Doctors urge more regulation for herbal treatments' *Brit Med J* (1998) **317**: p. 833

Inglis B, 'Fringe Medicine' (1964) Faber & Faber, London, p. 9

Lockley, GJ, Chief Fisheries Officer of New Zealand, Personal Communication.

Richmond, C. Personal Communication

Walrad R, (1960) 'The Misrepresentation of Arthritis Drugs and Devices in the United States'. Arthritis and Rheumatism Foundation, New York

Chapter 15

Gran JT and Skomsvoll JF, 'The outcome of ankylosing spondylitis, a study of 100 patients'. *Brit J Rheum.* (1997) **36**: pp. 766-71)

Le Fanu J, 'The Rise and Fall of Modern Medicine', Little, Brown and Company. (1999) p. 310

Radin EI, Paul IL and Rose RM, 'Role of mechanical factors in the pathogenesis of primary osteoarthritis' *Lancet* (1972) **i**: pp. 519-522

Acknowledgements

The following kindly provided helpful information through personal or telephone interviews:

Chapter 1. *The legacy from the past.*

Bywaters EGL, Hart FD, Glyn J, Scott JT, Spriddell P.

Chapter 2. *Academic development in the second half of the 20th century*

Hammersmith. Bywaters EGL, Scott JT, Hughes G.

Manchester. Kellgren JH, Sharp J, Jackson D, Jayson MIV.

Edinburgh. Hill AGS, Gardner D, Nuki G.

Chapter 3 *Other teaching hospitals in London.*
Yates DAH, Mathews J, Hughes GRV, Bywaters EGL. Graham R, Panayi G, Clarke AK, Hamilton EBD, Barnes CG, Thould AK, Axford J, Jenkins D, Wood PHN, Isenberg D, Edwards J.

Chapter 4 *Provincial Teaching Hospitals.*

Bristol: Cosh JA, Jayson MIV, Dieppe PA.

Birmingham. Bacon PA, McConkey B, Walton K.

Stoke Mandeville. Hill AGS.

Oxford, Mowat AG.

Cambridge. Hazleman B, Dingle J.

Liverpool, Williams. E.

Newcastle, Griffiths I, Cawston TE.

Leeds, Bird HA, Martin MFR, Emery P.

Sheffield, West H, Moll JMH, Russell RGG.

Cardiff. Lloyd KN, Jessop J, Davies J, Maddison PM. Williams G.

Aberdeen and Dundee, Reid DM.

Glasgow. Sturrock RD, Buchanan WW.

Belfast. Boyd W, Roberts SD.
I am particularly indebted to Prof Watson Buchanan who sent me enough material to fill a small book on the early life and times of the Centre for Rheumatic Diseases in Baird Street.

Chapter 5 *The Spa hospitals*

Harrogate. Bird HA, Martin MFR,

Droitwich. Popert J, Bacon PA.

Buxton. Sharp J, Kellgren JH.

Bath. Cosh JA, Clarke AK, Ring F, Collins AJ, Davies J.

Chapter 7 *Paediatric Rheumatology.* Ansell BM, Bywaters EGL, Woo P.

Chapter 8. *Surgical Rheumatology.* Kirkup J, Kellgren JH.

Chapter 9. *The Fourth Estate of Rheumatology*

Arthritis Research Campaign. Barnes C, Wood PHN, Andrews M.

Kennedy Institute. Gardner D, Scott JT, Hart FD.

Nuffield Foundation and Oliver Bird Fund. Hughes V and colleagues from the Oliver Bird Fund of the Nuffield Foundation, Kellgren JH.

Arthritis Care and Horder Homes. Woolf D.

The following patient groups in support of rheumatic disease sufferers kindly provided details of their work:
The Arthrogryposis Group. Piercy D.
Behçet's Syndrome Society. Seaman G.
British Sjögren's Syndrome Association. Ford M.
Ehlers-Danlos Support Group. Burrows V.
Lady Hoare Trust. Atkinson J.
Lupus UK. Hammer B.
Marfan Association UK. Rust D.
National Ankylosing Spondylitis Society. Rogers F.
National Assn. for the Relief of Paget's Disease. McCallum M.
National Back Pain Association. Montague N.
Perthés Association. Avery L.
Psoriatic Arthropathy Alliance. Chandler J.
Radar. Massie B.
Raynaud's and Scleroderma Association. Mawdesley AH.
Restricted growth Association. Rawlings H.
The Sarcoidosis Society. Cook A.
Skeletal Dysplasia Group. Wynne-Davies R.
The Scleroderma Society. Webster P.
The Scoliosis Association (UK). Harrison A.

Chapter 10 *The Science Base of Rheumatology.*

Panayi G, Jackson D, Bywaters EGL.

Chapter 13 *Complementary rheumatology, alternative rheumatology and the misrepresentation of drugs and devices*

Lockley GJ, (sometime Chief Fisheries Officer of New Zealand), Crompton J,

Chapter 14

The Patient's Story. Gooch E. (personal communication)

Acknowledgements to other works..

David Cantor has researched the history of the Arthritis Research Campaign up to the year 1970. Being allowed to see his work has considerably helped me. John Moll's 'The Heberden Society' has been a constant source of admiration for the excellence and thoroughness of his work. I could not hope to emulate it, but I have been helped by the detail about the early days of the Society. The two books published by the Royal Society of Medicine, George Kersley and John Glyn's 'A Concise International History of Rheumatology and Rchabilitation, Friends and Foes' and Geoffrey Storey's 'A History of Physical Medicine' have also been valuable sources, as has William Waugh's 'A History of the British Orthopaedic Association (ISBN 0 952184 0 X). Dr Gareth Jones gave me permission to quote from his book "The Aneurin Bevan Inheritance: the story of the Nevill Hall and District NHS Trust" (ISBN: 1 874538 17 4).

INDEX TO PLACES AND CONCEPTS

H

I

J

K

L

M

N

O

P

Q

R

S

T

U

W

Y

A

B

C